LAST DANCE

AT THE

SAVOY

ALSO BY KATHRYN LEIGH SCOTT

JINX FOGARTY MYSTERIES
Down and Out in Beverly Heels
Jinxed

FICTION
Dark Passages

NONFICTION
Dark Shadows: Return to Collinwood
The Bunny Years
Dark Shadows Memories
Dark Shadows Almanac
Dark Shadows Companion
Lobby Cards: The Classic Films
Lobby Cards: The Classic Comedies

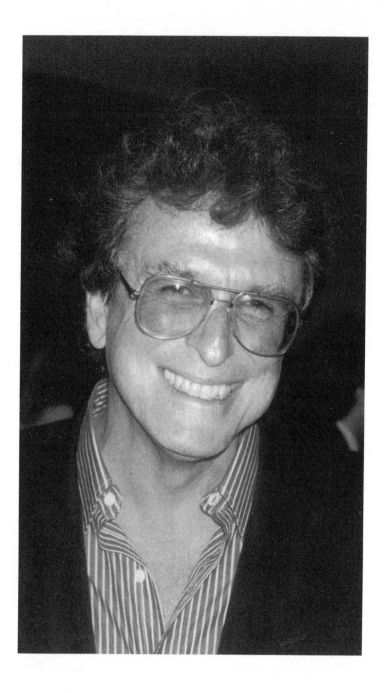

LAST DANCE

AT THE SAVOY

LIFE, LOVE AND CARING FOR SOMEONE WITH
PROGRESSIVE SUPRANUCLEAR PALSY

KATHRYN LEIGH SCOTT

Foreword by Yvette Bordelon, MD, PhD

Cumberland Press

New York

Photo credits: Chapter nine title: Joel Baldwin. Chapter ten interior: Ben
Martin. Chapter thirteen title: Joel Baldwin. Chapter twenty-one title:
Michael LeRoy. All other photos: Miller Family Archive.

Cover design by Nicholas Evans

Editing & formatting by Caitlin Alexander

Also available in e-book

E-book ISBN: 978-0-9862459-3-0

Trade paperback ISBN: 978-0-9862459-2-3

Library of Congress Control Number: 2016935348 / New Edition

Cumberland Press, New York, New York

For author contact and press inquiries, e-mail
cumberlandpressbooks@gmail.com. To order signed copies, visit
www.kathrynleighscott.com.

For Geoff and for everyone living with
prime-of-life diseases

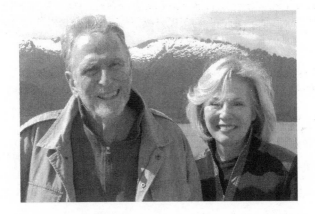

CONTENTS

FOREWORD

Last Dance at the Savoy is a beautifully written story of one couple's journey in dealing with the ravages of a rare neurological disease, progressive supranuclear palsy (PSP). While PSP is estimated to affect only five or six out of every 100,000 people, many more are affected by similar neurodegenerative diseases, including Alzheimer's and Parkinson's, which strike eleven out of 100 and two out of 100 people over the age of sixty-five, respectively. Related disorders include fronto-temporal dementia, amyotrophic lateral sclerosis (ALS, or Lou Gehrig's disease) and other prime-of-life diseases. In fact, as our population ages and as life expectancy increases, we will see a continued rise in cases of neurodegenerative disease. Almost everyone has experienced or will experience losing a loved one—spouse, parent, friend or relative—to one of these devastating disorders.

PSP is considered an atypical Parkinsonian disorder, also known as a Parkinson-plus disorder. This is because many features of PSP have commonalities with Parkinson's symptoms. Yet there are additional features (the "plus") that make PSP a distinctive disease. For instance, patients with PSP have severe, debilitating walking and balance problems, with falls occurring at the onset of the disease and becoming very frequent (sometimes daily) during the first several years. The other characteristic "plus" feature, for which the disease is named, is a gradual worsening of voluntary eye movements. Deterioration is subtle at first, affecting reading and vision, but leads to double vision and, eventually, to loss of eye movement altogether as the *supranuclear* (meaning above the area responsible for initiating and coordinating eye movements) part of the brain degenerates. *Palsy* means paralysis or loss of movement. And *progressive* refers to the relentless progression of not only those eye movement problems but also the many other symptoms of the disease. In contrast to Parkinson's disease, PSP progresses more rapidly and does not respond as well to medication.

PSP belongs to an additional category of diseases, frontotemporal lobar degeneration (FTLD). The FTLDs encompass a large number of neurodegenerative disorders characterized by varying degrees of cognitive and behavioral changes or impairment. Some of these diseases, including PSP, are related to abnormal accumulation of the protein tau in neurons in certain areas of the brain. For reasons that are not yet fully understood, tau, a protein responsible for critical functions in cells, starts becoming sticky and begins to abnormally fold, forming clumps in certain neurons that disrupt normal cellular function. Similar mechanisms are responsible for most neurodegenerative diseases, but they differ in the proteins that form those clumps (tau and amyloid in the case of Alzheimer's disease; alpha-synuclein in the case of Parkinson's disease).

PSP was first described in 1964 by Steele, Richardson and Olszewski. Since that time, there has been greater and greater recognition of the disease. Yet many patients are still misdiagnosed or experience significant delays in diagnosis because PSP is a rare disorder typically seen only by specialists or subspecialists in health care. In recent years, the pace of PSP research has accelerated dramatically, thanks to the efforts of numerous organizations formed to increase awareness of PSP and related disorders and to help fund research into treatments and therapies, and to the efforts of the many outstanding physicians and scientists around the world who have dedicated their lives to understanding and treating these diseases.

In the US, CurePSP has led this cause, growing significantly since its start in 1990. CurePSP provides resources and support for patients and families dealing with prime-of-life illnesses. The Tau Consortium, which has rapidly increased the pace of scientific discovery into the causes of tauopathies and the translation of those discoveries into meaningful treatments, has several PSP-related trials underway or planned. The list of ongoing research studies continues to expand, and up-to-date listings can be found on the CurePSP website as well as at ClinicalTrials.gov. Many other reputable organizations are listed in the resource guide at the end of this book.

With technological advances in genetics, imaging and other biomarker identification, we continue to make strides in generating better diagnostic tools and treatment strategies. In 2010, two clinical trials of novel medications were conducted in PSP subjects worldwide. For a disease so rare, and one recognized only fifty years ago, that is an amazing feat. While the medications were not found to be effective in PSP patients, the studies served as proof of the feasibility of future clinical trials. The dedication of patients, like Geoff Miller, and their families who are willing to participate in clinical research has resulted in immeasurable gains toward advancing our understanding of PSP and other neurodegenerative diseases.

From a personal perspective, the time that I spend seeing patients with PSP and related disorders is simultaneously extremely challenging and very rewarding. I am presented with many questions that are unanswerable: What caused this? Why me? Why did it take so long to receive a diagnosis? What will happen to me in six months? In one year? In five years? How can we slow the disease down? Why aren't there treatments that can help me? I am as frustrated by the lack of answers as my patients are. But during visits, I try to focus on the positive because *hope* is a very important ingredient in dealing with these diseases.

Talking to patients, I emphasize the treatments and interventions that are currently available and that we can try. Medication may provide some relief in certain symptoms for a period of time if there are no problematic side effects, but benefits vary enormously among patients. There is realistic hope, though, that some medications may help.

I also highlight the very positive role that nonmedication treatments play in maintaining quality of life: physical, occupational and speech therapy; daily exercise; counseling and cognitive-behavioral therapy; support groups; care-partner health and well-being; and additional care support in the home. There is realistic hope that these therapies will help.

Finally, we discuss research activities in the field, including current and upcoming clinical trials. I am most grateful for the willingness of patients and families to participate in research studies. It is through their generous contributions during life and, through brain donation, after that we have seen such significant progress in neurodegenerative disease research. Participation in clinical trials is not only enormously beneficial to those who will be affected by these diseases in the future; I find that it also significantly helps the person participating, who knows he or she is making this contribution to society. There is realistic hope that new treatments will become available as a result of such research.

Yet while I emphasize the positive and the hopefulness in dealing with prime-of-life diseases, at the same time I acknowledge the reality of the struggle, the frustration and grief. It is heartbreaking to watch someone gradually lose motor function and the ability to communicate while remaining cognitively intact and fully aware of the tragic consequences of his or her disease. It is humbling for me to see this. The impotence I feel is sometimes maddening. However, there is beauty amid the stressors, and I have watched couples and families unite and fight the illness with unfathomable amounts of grace and dignity and love.

Last Dance at the Savoy portrays this perfectly. By capturing the day-to-day and month-to-month changes that her husband experienced and how that shaped their lives and relationship, Kathryn Leigh Scott has crafted an extraordinary memoir that will resonate with those who have experienced the loss of a loved one to PSP and that will serve a source of guidance and inspiration for those currently dealing with this disease or a related disorder.

—

Yvette Bordelon, MD, PhD
Associate Clinical Professor
Department of Neurology
David Geffen School of Medicine at UCLA
January 2016

LAST DANCE

AT THE

SAVOY

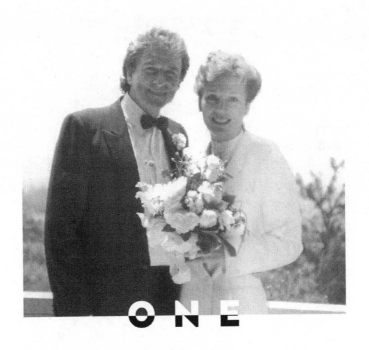

O N E

"NIGHT AND DAY"

On a warm midsummer's evening, Geoff and I strolled hand in hand across London's Waterloo Bridge after seeing a play at the National Theatre. Midway, we stopped to gaze across the Thames toward the Strand. At almost ten o'clock, the last glimmers of a startling sunset splashed the sky with flames of amber and crimson, casting a coppery glow on the spires of Big Ben and the

Houses of Parliament. I leaned into Geoff and he held me close, his cheek brushing my hair.

"There," Geoff whispered, nodding toward the shimmering windows of the Savoy Hotel. "That's where we'll have supper."

I squeezed his hand, then tilted my head back for a tender kiss. The Savoy was a perfect choice for our last romantic evening. We'd spent four blissful days and three nights filled with long walks, long lunches and lingering mornings, afternoons and evenings enjoying our time together and talking endlessly. We were still new to each other and savoring the melting euphoria of falling in love. I was in my forties but felt like a giddy teenager—and was behaving like one. I couldn't imagine a moment without Geoff, yet he was leaving on an early flight the following morning, returning to work publishing *Los Angeles* magazine. I would remain in England, filming on location. We wouldn't see each other again for weeks. I ached at the thought of it and pushed it from my mind, not wanting to spoil our last precious hours together.

As we turned off the Strand into the glittering entryway to the Savoy Hotel, I glimpsed the two of us mirrored in the silvery panels lining the curving walkway. In a fleeting cascade of images, I saw myself clad in a silky dress and strappy high heels, moving in step with Geoff, tall and handsome, his dark hair even curlier in the warm, moist air. He was wearing his new English blazer and the shirt and tie we'd bought for him that afternoon. I squeezed his hand, so proud to be with him.

We had no reservations for dinner, but we hovered only minutes before a maître d' ushered us to a table by a window aglow with lights sparkling along the river walk. Appropriately enough in this shrine to Art Deco, a string orchestra was playing Cole Porter. Geoff ordered champagne, then led me to the dance floor. We danced cheek to cheek to "The Way You Look Tonight," swaying in a gentle embrace, falling in love all over again.

I don't remember eating supper, although I know we had Dover sole. I barely remember drinking champagne, although it was my favorite, Veuve Clicquot. But I won't ever forget the intoxicating feel of Geoff caressing my bare shoulders, and the dizzying sense that I was floating in his arms as we danced to "They Can't Take That Away from Me."

In the pale light of morning, after a night of talking, touching and making love, there was only time for coffee and small spurts of scattered conversation. As Geoff finished packing his bag, I slipped a note into the pocket of his Burberry. We stood on the pavement hailing a taxi, holding hands, not wanting to let go, then kissed one last time before he climbed into a cab and was off. I stood hugging my arms in the morning chill, already missing him.

Back in my kitchen some few minutes later, I spotted Geoff's Burberry slung over the back of a chair. I grabbed the coat and raced back to the street, sure that he would realize he'd forgotten it and swing back. In that bygone era before cell phones there was no way to reach him. I stood at the curb, waiting, waiting—longing for him to return for one more fleeting moment. As the minutes dragged on and he didn't return, I pressed the coat to my face, breathing in his familiar scent, sad that he wouldn't be reading the message I'd slipped into the pocket.

—

Progressive supranuclear palsy (PSP) crept into our lives on cat's paws, insinuating itself without haste or fanfare. Looking back, there were early signs of its presence, but we couldn't have known it at the time. We mistook stiffening joints, forgetfulness, changes in vision, stumbles and even an occasional fall for nothing more than the vagaries of advancing years. There was no pain or suspicious shadow on an X-ray to alert us. There were no worrisome chronic conditions that couldn't be eased with Prilosec and a daily dose of prune juice. Until the falls became more frequent, more severe, and we came to realize something was wrong.

Had we been aware of Geoff's condition sooner, there was nothing we could have done about it except try to keep him safe from falls and injuries. The outcome was inevitable. Our way of dealing with the insidious, relentless advance of his rare neurological disease was to go on living with as little disruption as possible.

"No pain, no discomfort," Geoff would say when someone asked how he was doing. "I'm lucky. Could be worse."

Denial was the mechanism he found most useful in coping with the inexorable decline in his physical and mental condition. I was the one who trolled the Internet looking for information and assembling whatever we needed to adjust to fresh caregiving challenges. But together we took life a day at a time, not looking ahead except to book travel or plan dinner with friends. Geoff was always ready for a new adventure and nothing cheered him more than planning a trip.

On a starlit evening in April, more than two decades after our evening at the Savoy, I sat at Geoff's bedside, holding his hand, the air perfumed with the fragrance of yellow freesia blooming in a hanging pot outside an open window. Artie Shaw's "Night and Day" played softly, stirring memories. Geoff's eyes flickered. A smile curled the corners of his mouth. I leaned over, putting my hand to his shoulder, pressing my cheek to his. Breathing in his musky warmth, I felt the beat of my heart against his, our rhythms blending with the music as though we were dancing. *Should* be dancing!

My eyes burned and tears fell. I turned my head, letting the wetness seep into the pillow so Geoff wouldn't know I was crying. There was little we could hide from each other anymore, but if there was one thing we did want to keep from one another, it was tears. He didn't want to see them, and I didn't want grief to spoil whatever time we had left together.

I slid my hip over the metal railing of the hospital bed and eased myself into the narrow space next to Geoff, careful not to dislodge his oxygen tubes. The puffy green vinyl mattress, a motorized contraption installed to prevent bedsores, quivered with a gentle wheezing sound, adding its own rhythm to "Night and Day." Geoff sighed, murmuring something I could barely hear.

"I love you, too," I whispered. I matched my breathing to his and drifted off.

Sometime later, in his final hours, I sat holding his hand, my head on a pillow next to his, listening to CDs of his favorite music. I reminisced about his springtime jaunts to the Monterey Jazz Festival, an annual pilgrimage he preferred taking on his own. He'd head out the door in his worn jeans and tattered safari jacket, slide behind the wheel of his convertible and put the top down. While I stood hanging on the open car door, he'd load the CDs he'd specially selected for the drive. After a lingering kiss and a promise to call me en route, I'd stand back, waving goodbye until he pulled out onto the street.

He timed his departure perfectly so he'd arrive for lunch at the Cold Spring Tavern, an old stagecoach stop north of Santa Barbara that served buffalo burgers with beer on tap. Then, back on the road, he'd make it to Monterey in time to check in to a hotel and catch the first few sets of the Dixieland bands he loved. He'd call to let me know he'd arrived safely and then I wouldn't hear from him until he returned Sunday night, tired and ready for a martini and dinner.

"I used to give you my cell phone to take with you, remember? But you'd forget how to work it, or it would turn on accidentally in your pocket and I'd listen to your footsteps walking down the street. It was so maddening! But at least I knew you were all right, even if you couldn't hear me hollering at you, trying to get your attention."

I told him I was feeling a little like that now. I knew he was off on a journey, traveling alone. I didn't want him to go, but he couldn't let that stop him. "Somehow, when you get there, let me know you arrived safely. I'll miss you terribly, but we'll be together again. And I'll be fine. You've made me strong. Just save me a place."

Then, as Artie Shaw played Cole Porter, my fingertips brushed Geoff's cheek. His eyes opened, brilliant blue and clear. He looked so young, his skin taut and smooth, igniting memories of the man who had captivated me decades earlier.

"Do you remember? The orchestra played that piece when we danced at the Savoy?" Looking into his eyes, I hummed a bit of "Night and Day." "We danced to this and fell in love, remember?"

My lips to his ear, I whispered, "No tears. Not now. I'm with you as long as you need me. Then go and find a place for us."

The music of Artie Shaw and Cole Porter played on as I kissed Geoff's forehead, smoothed his hair and let him go where I couldn't follow, my memories still of being wrapped in his arms dancing at the Savoy.

If life is a miracle, so is death; the beginning and the end are both profound in their suddenness. Between the beginning and the end of our time together, the romance of getting to know each other and our last goodbye, I probably wouldn't change a thing, except to ask for more time.

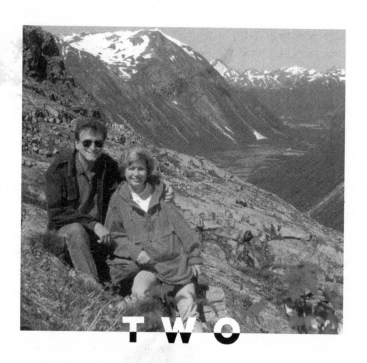

T W O

"YOUNG AT HEART"

Romance had found us at a transitional time in both our lives. Geoff, the founding editor of *Los Angeles* magazine, had recently shifted gears to become its publisher. I was a working actress, but my career focus had switched to writing and running Pomegranate Press, a small book-publishing company I'd founded in 1985.

We were both ripe for change. But frankly, when

Geoff unexpectedly came into my life again, I looked upon it as the resumption of an interrupted courtship of some twenty years.

We'd first met in New York in September 1968, shortly after the tumultuous political conventions, at a party hosted by Arthur Schatz, one of the photojournalists assigned to Richard Nixon's campaign. My boyfriend, *Time* magazine photographer Ben Martin, who'd been traveling with Nixon, had been reassigned to Hubert Humphrey's campaign. Ben was out on the hustings somewhere in the Pacific Northwest, and I hadn't seen him in weeks.

But I didn't mind his long absences too much because I was a busy young actress thoroughly wrapped up in my work. In June 1966, I'd been cast as Maggie Evans in the ABC Gothic daytime soap *Dark Shadows* and appeared in the show's first episode. With the introduction of Jonathan Frid as vampire Barnabas Collins, *Dark Shadows* had become a cult hit. By 1968, I was playing Josette duPrés, the doomed fiancée of Barnabas Collins, and enjoying every minute of our long days in the studio. My social life was essentially nil, other than quick drinks and supper after work with castmates at the Brittany du Soir, our favorite watering hole near the studio. Most of my evenings were spent learning lines and going to bed early.

However, it was the custom for all the wives and significant others (not a term used back then) of the journalists and photographers who were traveling with the campaigns to get together and party whenever a press contingent passed through New York. It was fun to hobnob with the very people one saw on evening newscasts. Most often these parties were held in someone's Kips Bay apartment on Thirty-Third Street near the East River, which seemed to be home base for an inordinate number of media people, including Ben. The two of us lived with a giant Maine Coon cat named Max in a one-bedroom apartment on the twentieth floor of the splendid I. M. Pei building.

Julian Wasser, a tall, skinny California-based photographer who was a colleague of Ben's, arrived at the party with two other men. I greeted them at the door and Julian introduced me to *Los Angeles* magazine editor Geoff Miller. Geoff was tall and boyishly slim, with dark, curly hair, and looked a bit like Clark Kent with his boxy, black-framed eyeglasses. I took in his warm smile and said hi, but my eyes quickly swung to the third man in the group, Tom Wolfe, resplendent in his trademark white suit. I recognized him immediately as the author of a book I'd just read, *The Electric Kool-Aid Acid Test*. I'd also read a piece he'd written for one of the first issues of *New York* magazine, which Clay Felker launched eight years after *Los Angeles* magazine.

I spent the rest of the evening talking with the trio. I quickly warmed to Geoff, who looked around at the beer-swilling gathering that included Ron Ziegler, Bob Haldeman and the rest of the motley Nixon crew and said, "This might be the worst frat party I've ever been to."

By the time the party broke up in the wee hours of the morning, Geoff and I were sitting by ourselves, knees touching, completely engrossed in each other. He was a forceful presence, with his resonant voice and powerful build, but his manner was gentle, effortless. We chatted easily, connecting on a deeper level than our breezy small talk would have indicated. I liked his

wit, humor and calm authority. I didn't want the evening to end.

Well past midnight, he reluctantly told me he had
to leave because he was catching an early flight back to
Los Angeles. We continued talking as I rode down in
the elevator with him. Once on the street, we decided
to have an Irish coffee together at a pub on the corner.
Our high-minded conversation (yes, books, philosophy
and Noble Solutions to the World's Ills!), leavened with
a good deal of laughter, barely concealed our budding
infatuation with each other. Eventually he hailed a cab
and that was that. I kept my secret crush on Geoff very
much to myself. After all, I had a boyfriend and Geoff
mentioned having a girlfriend. Besides, our lives were
so fixed on opposite coasts that I figured I would never
see him again.

But a couple of months later, I flew to Los Angeles
for a guest appearance on a television talk show. Once
again, I crossed paths with Geoff, this time in the company of his girlfriend, Barbara. The tall, stunning bru-
nette was working as both a *Time* magazine stringer and
an assistant to Joyce Haber, the famed *Los Angeles Times*
gossip columnist. My stay in Hollywood happened to
coincide with Hubert Humphrey's campaign swing
through town only days before the election. In an astonishing act of generosity, Barbara offered to drive through
rush hour traffic to the airport, with me following in my
rental car, so I wouldn't get lost trying to pick up Ben
when he arrived with Humphrey's campaign contingent. That weekend, Ben and I fell into a round of parties with other photographers and journalists and saw
quite a lot of Geoff and Barbara at various events.

Shortly after the election, Ben was posted to *Time*

magazine's Zurich and Paris bureaus, while I remained in New York doing *Dark Shadows*. Even though I ran into Geoff again on another trip to Los Angeles, any thought of kindling a romance was completely out of the question. While I was still attracted to him, both of us were involved in steady relationships. Besides, his magazine was based in Los Angeles and my television series was produced "live" in New York, so there was little temptation to embark on long-distance flirtation.

After filming *House of Dark Shadows* for MGM in 1970, I left the series and moved to Paris to join Ben. On July 3, 1971, Ben and I were married in a Midnight Sun wedding in the small Norwegian village that was my father's birthplace. Our family had also lived in that village for some time when I was a child, and our wedding served as an occasion for a huge family reunion. It also marked the emotionally significant restoration of the church bell, hidden in my uncle Olav's barn for the duration of the Nazi occupation, to a newly rebuilt belfry.

Following our wedding, Ben and I settled in London, taking up residence in a tiny 1790s cottage near Hyde Park that had once belonged to Henry Kaplan, one of the directors I'd worked with on *Dark Shadows*. For the next few years, Ben traveled as a photographer for *Time*, and I worked as an actress in film, theatre and television, including a six-month run in the West End doing *Harvey* with Jimmy Stewart. It was an exciting time for both of us.

In 1979, a role in a feature film brought me to New York, followed by an offer to do a television movie in Hollywood. I was then cast in several guest star roles in various series, which led to a lead role in the pilot of the

CBS television series *Big Shamus, Little Shamus*, with Brian Dennehy. The series was picked up and I remained in Los Angeles on my own until Ben eventually joined me several months later.

In one of those quixotic turns of events one can't quite believe, I found myself competing in a televised tournament called *Battle of the Network Stars* (*The Greatest Race*, anyone?), in which I ran, crawled, swam (none of it very well) and discovered what a kayak was. The upshot was that my team, led by that stalwart athlete Ed Asner, came in second, and I won enough money for a down payment on a dream house in the Hollywood Hills. Ben and I happily settled into the sweet bungalow that Jack Warner had once reputedly used as a *cinq à sept* for trysts with starlets. Ben continued to travel extensively for *Time*, and I found acting work that kept me busy in both Los Angeles and London. We maintained both our London cottage and the romantic little house, called Le Provençal, in the Hollywood Hills.

In the meantime, Geoff's fledgling magazine, with its city-centric lifestyle format, had spawned knockoffs in every major market in the nation. Geoff, who grew up in West Los Angeles, had designed the prototype for a literary magazine with cultural and service features while doing graduate work at UCLA. In June 1960, after earning his master's degree, he'd joined forces with Dave Brown, an advertising executive ten years his senior, to launch *Los Angeles* magazine in offices on the second floor of a building on North Rodeo Drive in Beverly Hills.

In 1973, Geoff and Barbara married and moved into a house in Benedict Canyon with Lori and Steve, Barbara's children from a previous marriage. Within a month of their marriage, Barbara was diagnosed with multiple sclerosis. For twelve years, Geoff ran the magazine, publishing weighty 600-plus-page issues, while nursing Barbara, whose condition never went into remission. She passed away in 1985.

By late 1987, my marriage to Ben was collapsing. Friends were astonished when we separated. "You seemed so happy, the ideal couple."

"He stopped traveling," I'd quip.

But the truth was we'd both gone our separate ways, which became evident when we spent more time together. Tellingly, when we lived in Paris during our first year of marriage, we spent only thirty-two days together. As he hopscotched around the world, we were left with little time to nurture the sort of family life I yearned for. Whenever I could, I would join him in some exotic locale, including a month-long photo safari in Africa for a *Time* cover story, but often Ben was in war zones and covering news stories. He loved his work, as I did mine, so when he was absent for months at a time, I immersed myself in writing and acting in Paris and London. I really couldn't complain, because my own life was fulfilling: I did a play at the Bristol Old Vic and made a film, *Providence*, in Paris with Alain Resnais, in a company that included Dirk Bogarde, Sir John Gielgud, Elaine Stritch and Ellen Burstyn. It was a thrilling time, but as enjoyable as my work was, travel and too much time apart took its toll on our relationship.

Our eventual divorce was amicable enough that we eschewed warring attorneys (and their fees), divided our stuff, helped each other pack up and parted without the lingering after bite of alimony. Unspoken was the knowledge that we'd always have one another's backs. Ben returned to his hometown in North Carolina and to the lovely antebellum house where he'd grown up. I remained in Los Angeles, working as an actress and writer. It was a painful separation for both of us, although we remained partners in Pomegranate Press. We also continued to share our beloved cottage in London.

In 1988, I'd written a coffee table book on film art that one of Geoff's editors selected for the magazine's December "Best Christmas Gift" feature. The editor proposed meeting him at the office prior to a lunch interview. On that fateful day, some twenty years after Geoff and I first met, he stopped by his editor's desk to congratulate me. We shook hands and I didn't want to let go. Nor, apparently, did he. We chatted for a few minutes while continuing to hold hands. He was still holding my hand as we walked out of the office and down the corridor to a waiting elevator. He didn't release my hand until the elevator doors began closing. I have no memory of my lunch with the editor. All I could think about was Geoff. I knew I couldn't bear to wait another twenty years to see him.

Fortunately I only had to wait another day. We had lunch together and things moved very quickly. A few months later, when I returned to England to shoot a television film, Geoff flew over for a long weekend that culminated in our evening dancing at the Savoy. It was while I was floating around the dance floor in Geoff's arms that I knew we would spend the rest of our lives together. And as that thought occurred to me, Geoff whispered in my ear, "I don't want to spend another day of my life apart from you."

Among the first things we discovered about each

other was our shared passion for travel. Geoff was envious that I'd trekked around Europe as a teenager and had spent several years living and working abroad. He wanted to make up for lost time, the many years when he and Barbara couldn't travel extensively because of her illness.

Travel became an intoxicating ingredient in our courtship. We seized every opportunity that came our way, much of it work-related. I went to Hawaii twice to film and Geoff flew over to spend long weekends with me. I got an assignment from a women's magazine to write about the reopening of the Dorchester Hotel in London, a trip that included a round-trip flight on the Concorde. Geoff was already booked on the press junket for *Los Angeles* magazine, which meant that we arrived together at the luxurious Park Lane Hotel, each registered in separate lavish suites. We visited his suite, then walked down the corridor to mine and tossed a coin to decide which we'd stay in.

Although it was a working trip for both of us, the five-day jaunt was a romantic getaway that included theatre, sightseeing and fine dining. We also strolled the short distance along Hyde Park to visit my cottage near Marble Arch, where a friend was staying.

On another occasion, I got an assignment from a travel magazine to do an article on the *Hurtigruten*, the Norwegian passenger and freight service that sails daily along the western coast from Bergen to the northern reaches of Kirkenes, a village on the Russian border. My mother joined us, which was helpful since she spoke Norwegian and could exercise her uncanny ability to engage almost anyone in conversation, particularly related to weather. We pulled into small villages along the route and, as mail and freight were loaded and new passengers boarded, we would disembark for a quick walk around the town. Aboard ship, Geoff marveled that "your people" had come up with so many resourceful ways to serve Jell-O and herring, though not (thankfully!) in combination.

In Vikebukt, my father's village, we partied with about twenty cousins by the light of the midnight sun on an island in the fjord below the family farm. Geoff was captivated by Ashild, one of my tall, beautiful cousins, who sat on a rock carving long, thin curls of salt-cured lamb, which we consumed with hardtack and malt whisky. For Geoff, the trip ranked as the most exotic holiday he'd ever had; for me, it meant going home again.

But among the most pleasurable travels were our frequent road trips close to home. Geoff was passionate about the splendors of California's beaches, deserts, mountains, vineyards and, most particularly, the rugged coastline. His favorite drive was Highway One, the coastal route through Monterey and Big Sur to Mendocino. Geoff kept clippings, brochures, maps and guidebooks in orderly files and annotated everything with his own comments and referrals. He liked nothing better than mapping out a route that would explore another hidden gem of natural beauty, a place of historical significance, a new restaurant or resort, a regional festival or music event—and most of these outings inspired articles in the pages of his magazine.

One of Geoff's editors commented that he worked for Geoff Miller, "who created a city magazine that tells you how to get out of town"—and thus was born the weekend guide, the annual restaurant guide and all the "50 Best" lists that were innovative at the time and became a staple of city magazines across the country.

In 1990, on one of our first trips to the Napa Valley together, Geoff and I were sitting on the terrace of the Auberge du Soleil, drinking champagne, when a cardinal in full crimson and white regalia walked onto the patio, gestured toward the magnificent sunset and playfully addressed the hotel guests: "Would anyone like to get married? I have a bit of time before the sun goes down."

Geoff leaped up and invited the priest to join us for a glass of champagne—and then asked him if he would marry us in six months. I don't know which of us was more surprised, but both the priest and I said yes! In one breathless moment, I was engaged, the priest booked and the wedding date set for late May. I was thrilled with Geoff's romantic spontaneity and quite pleased that a priest had agreed to marry us. Barbara was Jewish, I'm Protestant, and if Geoff, a Roman Catholic, had any hope of being married by a priest, he would have to settle for one of the Coptic variety.

The snowy-haired priest, who bore a vague resemblance to Pope John Paul, was indeed a cardinal in the Eastern Coptic church. He'd decided to become a priest at the age of seventy-two when his wife died. He told us that he'd divided his worldly possessions among his four grown sons, took a vow of poverty and claimed that afterward, "I never ate or drank so well in my life!" During the week, he ministered to the blind in San Francisco, and on weekends he traveled to the wine country to marry people. We exchanged phone numbers, shook hands, and he blessed us as we polished off the last of the champagne.

Geoff and I married in Napa Valley, California, on May 27, 1991, on the balcony of our suite at the Auberge du Soleil. Two bellboys were our witnesses, and the kindly priest helped button the back of my grandmother's vintage lace shirtwaist. I held a bouquet of sweet-smelling garden roses and we said our vows at sundown. After tipping the bellboys and ordering a second bottle of champagne for the priest before sending him on his way, Geoff and I stood on the balcony swaying in each other's arms, celebrating our future together.

If it's possible to encapsulate so many years, several lives and a lot of intricate passages, both exquisite and terribly painful, into a few pages, I'd like to think I've succeeded. Geoff and I courted and married, each for the second time. Ben, my former husband, eventually became our close friend, and we managed to share the use of the eighteenth-century cottage in central London that none of us could bear to give up. If I harbored any regrets about my life with Geoff, it was only that it had begun so late. How I would have loved raising a brood of children with him!

While our romance seemed like a fairy tale in the beginning, "happily ever after" didn't come as easily as "once upon a time." Several years into our life together, the loving, sweet-tempered man I married began lapsing into moody periods that I would later recognize as early signs of behavioral changes brought on by PSP. He brooded about constantly dropping things that seemed to slip out of his fingers. Picking them up again required too much effort and coordination, so he'd walk away, frustrated with himself. He'd rage when he couldn't find something that turned out to be within his reach, although he couldn't see it. "Stop moving things around where I can't find them!" he'd yell.

In turn, my heart would sink at the signs of one of these impending moods. I felt the pressure of accommodating him and avoiding anything that might annoy or frustrate him, such as a minor change in plans we'd made. I didn't balk when Geoff, who loved nothing more than writing on yellow legal pads, started asking me to tap in his words on my computer while he dictated. Reading his own handwriting had become difficult, but managing to do his own typing even more impossible.

Meanwhile, my internal voice kept questioning: What's all the fuss about? Why can't he just pick it up, put it away? Why do drawers always stick when he tries to close them? Why is it my fault that he can't find the peanut butter in the cupboard? His outbursts were unpredictable, but always over something trivial, and seemed to come in cycles. All was well for long periods, then abruptly there would be days of sullen moods and bad temper.

In my lighter moments, I put these rocky times down to a "Mars vs. Venus" thing, two different planets awkwardly revolving around each other in a strange solar system known as marriage. If only I'd registered then that we might be dealing with symptoms of a neurological disease, we could have spared ourselves considerable marital strife and woe.

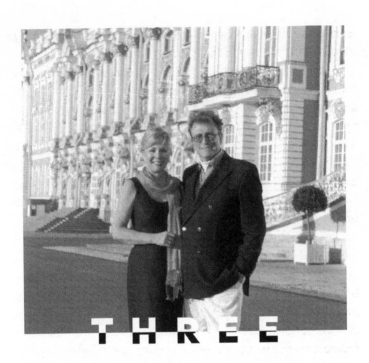

THREE

"AROUND THE
WORLD"

Life was sweet in the spring of 2007. After almost sixteen years of marriage, our dance cards were filled with travel, a busy social calendar and work that gave each of us pleasure. I'd finished a draft of a novel and was researching an article for *Opera News*. Geoff had long since retired from *Los Angeles* magazine, but occasionally did some consulting work. Aside from a few hours during the day when we went out on our own, we spent much of our time together. We each had an office at home, both of them upstairs at opposite ends of the house. Geoff usually went out for lunch, but we dined together every evening, often with friends, and rarely spent time apart.

One of those times apart occurred that spring when Geoff attended the Monterey Jazz Festival, driving there by himself. I remained in Los Angeles to film a television commercial. I missed him, but we had a trip coming up, and I spent my evenings preparing for our departure the following week.

We'd planned an ambitious six-week itinerary that would take us from Los Angeles to Minneapolis, New York, London and a side trip to Italy to celebrate our wedding anniversary. I'd already arranged for our close friend Harry Hennig, who is a private detective, to stay in the house while we were gone. Harry invariably drove us to the airport and picked us up on our return, a favor we never took for granted.

The only thing out of the ordinary about the start of that trip was that for the first time I did the packing for both of us. Geoff had always packed his own suitcase, but lately I'd noticed he was choosing clothing haphazardly. He became irritable if I suggested more appropriate items, so I avoided commenting unless it was absolutely necessary. Without giving it much thought, I did what married people do—I pitched in, picked up the slack, accommodated—and tried to do so without a tiresome squabble. And clothing wasn't the only issue.

"You never used to find fault with everything I did,"

he'd say. "I can't help it if I'm growing old. Consider the alternative!"

I'd laugh because Geoff was funny even when he was annoyed. His sense of humor masked such a lot, but I could also see his growing frustration. Zippers were always getting stuck, and he had difficulty with snaps, buttons and laces. He preferred pullover shirts and slip-on shoes, whatever was easy. He may have sensed his body was beginning to betray him, but it would have been his nature to admit to nothing more than advancing years slowing him down—and make light of it.

If anything, Geoff found comfort in those advancing years. His father, an executive with Union Carbide, had died at the age of sixty-three, just as Geoff completed grad school at UCLA and was launching *Los Angeles* magazine. His mother had passed away after a stroke at age sixty-one. Brother Ed, six years older and unwell for many years, died of diabetes complications shortly after his seventieth birthday. From all appearances, Geoff, who drank moderately, never smoked and ate a healthy diet, seemed strong and vital for his years.

At age sixty-nine, he was tall, handsome and robust, with broad shoulders, a strong grip, an easy smile and a deep, resonant voice. He could deliver a zinger with expertise and ease contentious dinner party conversation with gentle humor that slighted no one. His warmth captivated everyone, certainly me—and even Ben, my first husband, although I prayed they weren't indulging in too many chummy can't-live-with-her-can't-live-without-her conversations when they got together. Indeed, life was sweet.

By the time Geoff returned from the Monterey Jazz Festival, our bags were packed. Our first stop was

Minneapolis to visit my family. With both my mother and Aunt Pat in their early nineties, we were making frequent trips to visit them.

My mother had recently begun using a walker. It made her feel more secure, although she could still walk quite well on her own. She also wore a hearing aid despite strong evidence she could overhear private conversations through closed doors and concrete walls. Other than a bothersome swollen gland in her neck, she appeared to be in excellent health. She was still quick-witted and fully capable of cooking meals, programming a VCR and driving her car through a Minnesota blizzard. Her life was full with my two brothers and their families living close by and her involvement with church and Norwegian cultural activities. And she liked to shop.

Aunt Pat, two years younger than my mother, lived in her own apartment in the same senior living facility, a sprawling, beautifully landscaped complex that looked like a country club. In fact, this senior co-op was the handsomely converted elementary school my brother and I had attended. My mother and aunt lived completely separate lives, but after my aunt's eyesight began to fail, my mother would invite her for meals and take her grocery shopping. These two highly independent, opinionated women, who never quite got along, shared a fervent passion for The Young and the Restless. I once overheard them making lurid comments about someone's complicated love life before I realized they were talking about soap opera characters.

It was while we were all walking out onto my mother's patio one afternoon that I realized my husband was actually less steady on his feet than either my mother or my aunt. It wasn't the first time I'd noticed Geoff had trouble getting out of his chair or putting a glass down on a table. But now his difficulties were so pronounced that my mother commented on it. Geoff's gait was slower than theirs, and he was more than twenty years younger than either of them. He moved even more unsteadily when he tried to carry something in his hand, such as a book or a cup.

My aunt, who at times exhibited stupefying candor, watched Geoff make his way to the patio and commented, "You're gonna be needin' a walker yourself pretty soon." We laughed, but both women winced every time Geoff sat down heavily. "You're plopping," my aunt would tell him. "You'll break a chair one of these days." My mother, I noticed, served him lemonade in a plastic tumbler rather than using one of her good glasses.

Geoff didn't appreciate what he considered their constant criticism. He was only too happy when we boarded our flight to New York a few days later.

Geoff loved New York and had always looked forward to his business trips to Manhattan. I'd studied acting in New York and spent the first seven years of my career working in the city. When Geoff retired from the magazine in 1994, I suggested we look for a little pied-à-terre. "All we need is something the size of a junior hotel suite," I said.

We found old friends in Los Angeles and Connecticut with the same idea—and we all knew another couple with a house in Upstate New York, who happened to have an apartment in the city that they seldom used. We all shook hands on a deal that allowed us to split costs on a spacious, rent-stabilized apartment on the Upper East Side. We ended up sharing Barry and Beth's two-bedroom, two-bath apartment with our close friends Joel, Hannah, Douglas and Francoise for several years, managing at least five business and pleasure trips a year to New York. On most visits we had the apartment to ourselves. Occasionally we'd overlap with one of the other couples occupying the second bedroom. It was a perfect arrangement, but it made us hunger for a place of our own.

On one of our trips in 2001, a friend in real estate insisted we look at a newly renovated studio apartment on Fifty-Second Street near the East River. As we walked toward the building, I could see Geoff taking in the quiet residential cul de sac, with its Art Deco architecture. He claimed afterward that he "bought" our apartment before seeing it. In those first haunting weeks after the 9/11 terrorist attack, Geoff embraced the incredible spirit of New Yorkers and wanted a tangible stake in being part of the city's recovery.

Within a month we returned to New York, this time driving a U-Haul cross-country with basic furnishings for our new apartment. I bought Geoff a trucker's cap, and he plotted out a scenic route that was certainly not the shortest distance between Los Angeles and Manhattan. In fact, Geoff couldn't resist veering off the main highway every time he saw a sign touting a scenic view, historical site or an old mining town—we even toured the Hershey's chocolate factory in Pennsylvania and watched candy kisses rolling down a conveyor belt. We avoided the big cities and generally stopped for the night in college towns, on Geoff's theory that with visiting parents there would be good food and lodging. Like Lucy and Desi, we encountered our share of mishaps and bad weather driving cross-country, but it was also great fun. Not surprisingly, it took almost three weeks before we pulled up at our apartment building in New York City.

Since our building, designed by architect Emory Roth, had been constructed in 1930, only one tenant had lived in our large, ground-floor studio apartment. Bob was his name. He was an actor, former OSS agent and well-known raconteur and bachelor-about-town, who threw lots of parties. When the building went co-op, Bob remained a tenant. His apartment, according to the doormen, was not redecorated in the entire time he lived there. He'd had a standard-issue, dome-top Kelvinator and other prewar kitchen fixtures that had never been updated. The apartment, when we bought it, had been completely gutted and renovated, but it retained all the charm of its original architectural features. We loved it, and scoured the city for Art Deco furnishings and fixtures.

We both preferred living on the ground floor, especially me, with my dislike of elevators. Geoff liked the idea of reading the newspaper and looking up to see people walking by on the street outside our windows. We were both so used to leaving the doors of our house open to the garden in Beverly Hills that we occasionally left our apartment door ajar. More than once, other residents in the building would step inside and say, "Looks like Bob's having another party!"

One of Geoff's great joys was walking the city streets. He knew the bus and subway lines as well as any native New Yorker. He loved stopping in at one of his many jazz haunts, particularly Birdland on West Forty-Fourth Street. He wouldn't miss the Gully Low

Jazz Band on Wednesday afternoon, or Big Band on Fridays. Geoff's knowledge of jazz was encyclopedic. At Birdland, the best musicians in New York (Geoff would say the world) would play for two hours, starting at 5:15, before heading off to work in the Broadway pit orchestras and other concert venues around town. Geoff liked getting to Birdland early and securing a seat at the bar. James, the bartender, knew him by name and served him draft beer and plates of jambalaya. For two precious hours, he'd sit entranced, listening to great jazz played by musicians sight-reading complex charts. Sometimes I would join him, but most of the time Geoff went to Birdland by himself.

Often he would leave in the morning and spend an entire day exploring various New York neighborhoods, occasionally calling me in the late afternoon to join him for an early dinner in some new spot he'd found in Greenwich Village or Chelsea. One evening we had dinner at the River Café in Brooklyn, then went next door to the Barge to hear jazz. Afterward, we walked across the Brooklyn Bridge to catch a First Avenue bus back home to our apartment. Schiller's Wine Bar in the East Village (where the table wine was designated "cheap," "decent" and "good") and Pastis in Soho were favorite dining spots. Occasionally we'd take the subway to an art gallery opening in Lower Manhattan and have dinner in the neighborhood, or take a bus to the Ninety-Second Street Y for music or a lecture.

But during the two weeks we were in New York in the spring of 2007, there were several occasions when I noticed Geoff had difficulty walking. Boarding buses had become a challenge. He'd climb one step and start to fall backward. I'd grab his arm or give him a push from behind. There were some alarming occasions when he almost toppled back on me, but we'd laugh them off.

"Kneeling buses" were to blame, Geoff would say. "You're left standing at a slant on the top step when you're trying to put your pass in the machine." I'd agree.

One day he arrived back at the apartment and told me he'd slipped on the sidewalk. "I was flat on my back," he said, "and several people reached out to help me up. Where else but New York would people give you a hand!"

Later that night, when we were getting ready for bed, I saw a dark bruise on his hip. "You must've fallen hard," I said. "Are you okay?"

"Nothing broken," he said. "Nothing to worry about."

While I was preparing dinner one evening, Geoff went to the corner store to get milk for breakfast. I was peeved he took such a long time on a simple errand when he knew I would be waiting to serve dinner. I looked out the window and spotted him walking unsteadily, a milk carton about to tumble out of the plastic bag he was carrying by one handle. The doorman hurried to give him a hand.

"Where were you?" I asked, when he finally reached the apartment. "Did you stop in at Billy's for a drink on the way?"

"No," he snapped. "Get the milk yourself next time."

More than once, when he tottered home in the early evening, I'd accuse him of having a drink too many. Often his speech was slurred, but he would insist he'd only had a beer at a jazz club—then get angry because

I'd criticized him. Sometimes I'd hear the scratching of his key trying to unlock the door. I'd open the door myself and glare at him. He'd glare back because he knew what I was thinking.

"If I want to have a drink, I'll have one."

"Fine, but one drink doesn't make you tipsy!"

"I'm not drunk!"

"Then why are you wobbling? You can't even unlock the door!"

"Leave me alone!"

"But it's not safe. You could fall crossing the street."

And so it would go. Sharp words. Accusations. Anger and frustration followed by long, sullen silences. But I knew he wasn't drinking more than usual. And just as often I would notice him slurring words and losing his balance when he'd had nothing at all to drink. I had a gnawing sense that something was wrong and began feeling anxious when Geoff was gone for long periods on his own.

By the time we flew to London in May, I was aware that Geoff was having difficulty not only handling luggage and climbing stairs, but even dressing himself. Buttons and zippers, or anything that required two hands, aggravated him. He hung on to the sink with one hand while brushing his teeth or filling a glass with water. He would only wear blue jeans, but often left the top button undone. He decided to grow a beard rather than shave. Now that I'd started looking for these signs, I saw them in everything he did, and it made me even more anxious.

Although I had not lived in London full-time for several years, I still considered it "home" and always looked forward to our visits. But the Cottage, built in 1791, had always required some tricky maneuvering on the steep, curving staircase and in the narrow spaces in the small upstairs bedrooms. Now the house had become something of an obstacle course for Geoff. The deep, old-fashioned bathtub and low couch and armchairs with soft cushions were a challenge. As much as he loved the Cottage, and its proximity to Hyde Park, I could see that some things had become an ordeal for him. I also noticed that as much as Geoff enjoyed the London newspapers, he only bothered to read the front page. It had become hard for him to turn pages.

Since Geoff's retirement, we had visited London at least twice a year and used the house as a hub for excursions to Paris, Dublin, Prague, St. Petersburg and elsewhere in Europe. On this trip, we'd planned a side trip to Italy. I'd booked the two-hour Ryanair flight to Bologna three months earlier at a cut-rate fare of eleven dollars each, including tax. Deep into our middle years, Geoff and I had reverted to our youthful hippie ways and means, pursuing adventure at bargain prices. We'd already made similar cheap-fare excursions on Ryanair and easyJet and enjoyed the trips. I was more apprehensive this time, but we both looked forward to the adventure.

The words "explore strange new worlds" and "boldly go where no man has gone before" had looped through my brain since our journey to Bologna, Italy, began with a predawn, hour-long coach trip from Central London to Stansted Airport. In 1942, the U.S. Air Force had constructed an airfield on the site of a 2,000-year-old Roman burial ground. The rural airstrip had since expanded into England's third-largest airport, boasting a vast space-age terminal apparently designed for humanoids with a taste for molded plastic and little need of creature comforts. After navigating various chutes and shuttles, we'd been herded aboard the no-frills Ryanair flight.

The primary reason those Gene Roddenberry phrases were floating around my mind was that I'd been invited to attend STICCON as a celebrity guest at the annual meeting of Italy's Trekkies. Two young people, both Star Trek fans, were waiting to greet us at Forlì Airport; their mission, to deliver us to the seaside town of Bellaria, the site of the festivities. The earnest-looking man behind the wheel of a miniature Fiat was an accountant. The red-haired woman, who loaded our two small carry-ons into the car's miniscule trunk, worked as a travel agent. Both were in their late twenties and shyly eager to meet, in person, the actress who had played Nuria in the "Who Watches the Watchers" episode of *Star Trek: The Next Generation*.

Sleepy, hungry and achy from what already seemed like a long journey into deep space, I nevertheless tried to present myself as the stalwart, *sympathique* figure I'd portrayed on the small screen some fifteen years earlier. But without the prosthetic forehead and pointy green ears that makeup man Mike Westmore had laboriously applied every morning, I bore no resemblance whatsoever to the fierce, primitive creature from a distant planet that I'd once played. Instead of Nuria's long black braids, my blond hair was pulled into a ponytail under a wide-brimmed straw hat, and I was wearing jeans with a cotton shirt.

"I'm not looking much like a Mintaken this morning," I said when the young man approached.

"Oh, Miss Scott, I would have recognized you anywhere!" he said, prompting us all to laugh.

As we settled ourselves in the back seat of the car, I related a story I'd often told about Geoff joining me for lunch in the studio commissary on one of the few days we were filming on a sound stage at Paramount instead of on location. I'd walked into the large, airy dining room and approached Geoff, who was waiting near the entrance. He didn't recognize me at all, not even when I called his name. He turned around, looking for me, even though I was standing directly in front of him. I thought he was teasing me before I realized he really didn't recognize me under the wig and elaborate makeup. Throughout our lunch he'd stared at me, not believing I could be so transformed. I figured I'd be telling that story, among others, a few more times that weekend.

While we drove through the picturesque countryside, I answered questions about the *Star Trek* episode while Geoff gazed out the window. So far, so good, I thought. We were both excited about the trip to Italy because the STICCON event coincided with our sixteenth wedding anniversary. We'd made plans to stay in a luxury hotel in Venice following our weekend with the Trekkies.

After we checked into our hotel room in Bellaria, we stood on our balcony, looking out on the smooth gray waters of the Adriatic. The scene had the old-fashioned charm of a vintage seaside postcard. Gaily striped cabanas lined the seashore, with canvas deck chairs set out in neat rows across the smooth sand. Bellaria, an ancient fishing village, had become a seaside resort with quaint village streets open to pedestrians only. Vehicles were restricted to the waterfront road running along the perimeter of the town.

As tired as we were after the long journey, we thought the day was too beautiful, the seaside too inviting, to spend our time napping. Instead, we decided to walk on the beach before returning to the hotel for a late lunch. Off we went, both of us barefoot, with Geoff wearing bathing trunks and a tee shirt. I was in a bikini and light cotton shift.

The midday sun was hot and the sand burned our feet. We made our way to the water's edge and waded through the cool, gentle surf toward an old metal pier. The structure was painted pale blue, with sparkling objects that appeared to be lanterns dangling from the railings. I reached the pier first and turned back to tell Geoff to duck his head. He did, but not soon enough.

He knocked his head and fell backward into the shallow water. We both laughed and I splashed over to help pull him to his feet. We even laughed when blood trickled down his face. But then he lost his footing and slipped back into the surf, looking a bit dazed. Within moments, his face, neck and eyeglasses were covered in blood, staining the seawater red. I knelt next to him, cupping water in my hands to wash away the blood.

A burly sunbather rushed to our aid, speaking Italian. We laughed and waved him away, with Geoff insisting he wasn't badly hurt.

"Just a bump," he said. "You know how head wounds bleed."

But with blood oozing down his forehead, dripping off his nose onto his teeth and into his ears, I grew alarmed. The sunbather looked at Geoff in horror and began tugging at his arm.

"Just get me back to the hotel and under the shower," Geoff said, trying to stand up.

By now, we'd attracted a small crowd, everyone offering us small tissues and helping hands. I gestured toward our hotel and took Geoff by the arm. The crowd, now even larger, stopped us. I smiled again and tried to move ahead. Arms went up, blocking our way. A lifeguard pushed through the crowd, gesticulating and sputtering a stream of Italian. I caught a word that sounded like "hospital."

"No, no," we both said, and tried to work our way toward the hotel.

A vehicle pulled up, the doors were opened, and we were both firmly inserted into the business end of the Tonka-toy-size village ambulance. I wrapped my arms around Geoff, supporting him as we huddled together, smiling and calling out *grazias*, until the doors were closed. In less time than it takes to swallow an espresso, we were whisked through town and deposited in front of a small white building. We stood like strangers in paradise, gazing at the entrance to a pristine, eerily silent and seemingly uninhabited clinic.

We entered and stood for a moment, both of us now covered in blood, wondering if perhaps hospitals in Italy closed for lunch. We turned to leave, but stopped at the sound of a gentle female voice saying, "*Prego.*"

The voice belonged to a beautiful, bright-eyed young woman wearing crisp white scrubs. Her long, dark hair was pulled into a thick ponytail. Walking up behind her was a tall, handsome young man in matching white scrubs. Geoff and I stood clutching each other—two half-dressed, middle-aged, blood-soaked Americans who had wandered in off the street with no identification, money or Blue Cross cards, facing off with Italian Barbie and Ken versions of nurse and doctor. The woman smiled and gestured for us to follow them. We entered an examining room and quickly learned that Barbie and Ken were both doctors and both spoke English.

Geoff was helped onto an examining table and given a thorough wash with antiseptic. The wound was examined and a circular patch of hair was shaved off his crown. He looked like Friar Tuck. Amid gentle teasing and laughter, he was stitched up and given a tetanus shot. I smiled and held his hand throughout, but despite my outward calm, the sight of Geoff lying on the gurney, his face gray and bloodstained, left me deeply shaken. We were so far from home and "the big guy" looked so frail and vulnerable. How could strong, solid, broad-shouldered Geoff be so easily knocked off his size-eleven feet? These thoughts roiled through my mind as I stood watching him get patched up. Would they keep him in hospital?

No, to my surprise, we were to be sent on our way. I had imagined that with a head injury, Geoff might at least have to spend a few hours in the infirmary for observation. Instead I was presented with an ice pack to hold on Geoff's head. We laughed some more as Geoff caught sight of himself in a wall mirror and exclaimed, "I look like the return of the living dead!"

We'd had such fun that, as we were leaving, it occurred to us to invite our gorgeous doctors to dine with us that night. They declined, but it also occurred to us how odd it was that they'd asked only for Geoff's full name in order to write a prescription. We hadn't been asked for identification, much less payment for services. Our doctors walked us back to the entrance and, in an-

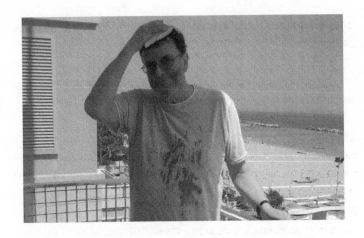

other Rod Serling moment, stood framed in the clinic's doorway waving goodbye to us as we walked out into the hot afternoon sun.

It then dawned on us that we would have to walk back to the hotel and we had no idea where it was. Geoff clamped the ice pack on his head, I took his arm, and together we set out, barefoot and bloodstained, in search of our seaside hotel. We hadn't walked more than a block when we heard music. As we turned a corner, a marching band rounded another corner at the far end of the street. It was, eerily enough, a funeral cortege. Two young women carried a basket of gladiolas between them, followed by women in black surrounding a cart with a casket pulled by men in hats and black suits. Out of respect for the deceased and loved ones, Geoff and I stopped in our tracks as the procession passed by. Needless to say, every eye turned to take us in.

"I probably look worse than the corpse," Geoff whispered. Somehow we managed not to crack so much as a smile.

"This is totally surreal," I said, whispering despite the blare of brass, drums and accordion music. "Who would believe us?"

"Fellini," Geoff said. "He came from Rimini, the next town down the coast."

We followed the smell of the sea back to our hotel, stopping along the way at a street vendor to buy Geoff an Italian student cap to cover his bandaged head. The cheap black cotton cap looked so good on him, I bought two extras.

But as we walked toward our hotel, I had a nagging sense that the mishap couldn't be blamed on fatigue, glare off the ocean or any of the other reasons we'd come up with. Back in our room, we stripped off our blood-soaked clothes, dumped them in the bidet filled with cold water and took a hot shower together.

As I soaped the blood staining Geoff's chest, I wondered how he could not have ducked enough to avoid cracking his head on a bolt that was so visible? The underside of the pier wasn't that low. But I was also feeling guilty that I hadn't somehow prevented it from happening. Why hadn't I foreseen the danger? I should have protected him, made sure he ducked his head. Lately, I always seemed to be on the alert for anything that might cause Geoff to stumble or lose his balance, so why had I slipped up this time? Usually I would grip his arm when we were climbing stairs or walking on uneven surfaces. If he did hurt himself, I would find some excuse to account for it. This time I couldn't.

On a trip to London in 2006, Geoff and I had taken the Underground back to the Cottage after attending a matinee. We'd gotten separated on the escalator when a rush of schoolchildren scrambled between us. Geoff lost his balance and fell backward. By the time I reached him, two other passengers had helped him to his feet. He had a bad cut over his eye and scrapes on his arm. Within minutes, a transit guard called paramedics and we were hustled into an ambulance on our way to St. Thomas' Hospital. Some seven hours later, Geoff was released with his arm in a sling and his head bandaged. We took a taxi home and blamed Geoff's misfortune on rambunctious school children. Of course, the mishap didn't stop us from continuing to ride the Underground, but we reminded ourselves to be more careful.

We also continued riding the double-decker London buses even after another perilous incident when Geoff lost his footing on the top deck and fell backward down steep stairs. I screamed, terrified he'd been badly injured. Instead, he was lying in a heap at the foot of the stairs, a grin on his face, insisting he was fine. Other passengers looked on, horrified, as two young men got him back on his feet and, at Geoff's insistence, helped him climb back up to the top deck. Few things delighted Geoff more than sitting in those coveted top-deck front seats. He wasn't about to give them up because of a little stumble down the stairs.

Back in our seaside hotel, I took stock of our situation while Geoff napped. We still had several more weeks of travel ahead of us, taking trains, buses and the Underground. Aside from our three days in Bellaria, we would be visiting familiar old haunts in Bologna, Venice and London. We were accustomed to cobblestone streets, narrow stairs and the eccentricities of ancient plumbing, yet I worried that it had all become too much of a challenge for Geoff.

We'd booked a beautiful suite in a grand old hotel in Venice for our anniversary, but once we got there I saw disaster looming at every turn. I glanced at the bathtub and knew we wouldn't be enjoying a luxurious soak together.

"It would take a crane to get me in and out of there," Geoff said, and laughed.

I laughed, too. But a shiver raced through me as I took in the steep sides of the tub, the slippery old marble and the lack of any grip bars, or even a handy bath rail. We showered together for the romance of it, as well as to satisfy my unspoken concern that he could slip and fall without my support. I insisted Geoff hang on to the faucets while I soaped him down.

We didn't walk around as much as we normally did in Venice, but we'd already seen most of the sites. We sat in cafés instead. Fortunately we'd traveled with only carry-on luggage and I was able to shoulder both pieces myself while still managing to grip Geoff's arm. On the flight home, Geoff mumbled, "I'm not as young as I was," as we eased ourselves into the cramped Ryanair seats. Then we laughed. Because, really, every concession we had to make seemed funny to us. And as long as we laughed together, everything was fine.

Besides, Geoff was game for more travel and suggested we think about taking a cruise from Venice to the Greek Isles sometime soon. I told him I'd look into it.

When we returned to London, my first call was to my oldest friend in England, Dr. Christine Pickard, a National Health GP and medical journalist, who also served as a forensic doctor on twenty-four-hour police emergency calls. Who better to turn to in our time of need? I invited Christine and her husband, Gordon, a filmmaker and antique-camera collector, for dinner and told her about Geoff's head injury.

"Geoff took a spill in Italy and has stitches in his scalp that have to come out within ten days," I said. "Are you up for it?"

"Of course," she said. "Have you got rubbing alcohol and tweezers, or do I need to bring a kit?"

I had the medical supplies on hand, and also the makings for Geoff's favorite English summertime drink, a Moscow Mule. Geoff never failed to mention that the Moscow Mule had been invented at the Cock and Bull pub on the Sunset Strip—though, oddly, ginger beer, the primary ingredient besides vodka, was only readily available in England. We sat in the garden at a table under the cherry tree and sipped our Moscow Mules while Christine set to work on Geoff's skull.

"Nice job," Christine said, inspecting the stitches, tweezers in hand. "Bellaria, you say?"

We told our story about Barbie and Ken. We all laughed, Geoff more than anyone. "Never hurt a bit," he kept saying.

Very late that night, the phone rang. It was my mother calling from Minneapolis.

"I hope I didn't wake you," she said, in a voice that made her words no more than a formality. "I was wondering if you could come home."

"Of course. When?"

"Now. I really want you home with me."

"What's wrong, Mom?" I asked, knowing instinctively what I would hear.

"That swollen gland turns out to be lymphoma. It's cancer. I've decided not to have any treatment." There was a pause before she added, "If it costs a lot to change your tickets, I'll cover it."

I swallowed hard and dealt with the easy matter first. "Thank you, but I'll take care of it. We'll be back as soon as I can arrange a flight."

It was just like my mother to avoid drama in dealing with big issues. She saved it for the small stuff. I'm pretty sure I'm my mother's daughter in that respect. I glanced at Geoff, who was still tucked in bed. "I love you, Mom. I'll change our tickets and get back to you."

"I want you here soon. I don't have a lot of time."

"I know. I understand. I'm sorry, Mom. Are you feeling okay now?"

She knew what I meant. "We can talk about everything when you get here."

I called the airline and rebooked before climbing back into bed. My stomach was in knots. I spent a sleepless night mulling over the swift changes happening in our lives. The signs posted in public spaces came to mind: *If you see something, say something.*

But the difference between an ordinary mishap or a lingering sore throat and the warning signs of something more serious seem obvious only in hindsight. When my mother told me that lymphoma was the cause of the swollen gland in her throat, an image sprang to mind of seeing her finger the lump below her ear, then touching the other side of her neck where there wasn't a lump. She'd mentioned how odd it was that the discomfort she felt was on only one side of her neck. Why hadn't I questioned it; urged her to see a doctor? If I had, could the malignancy have been caught at an earlier stage?

Looking back now, I realize Geoff had exhibited signs of a neurological disorder long before I recognized the changes in his behavior as a cause for concern. In fact, with the eagle eye of hindsight, I can recall mild tics, mannerisms and peculiar responses that seemed only a little odd some ten years before diagnosis. He would tap surfaces before setting something down. He invariably failed to close the left door of a cupboard. He would become annoyed when I tried to draw his attention to something to his right or left. His fingers would move to adjust his eyeglasses, even when he wasn't wearing them. At the time, I considered such behavior annoying, amusing or mildly eccentric, but certainly not worrying.

In our daily life, I didn't notice how much I was accommodating, making excuses, picking up the slack when Geoff faltered, because it's what one naturally does living with a spouse or family member. I cleaned up spills, swept up breakage and took his arm when he stumbled, without really taking note of how commonplace these occurrences were becoming. His seeming indifference, bouts of anxiety and harsh outbursts were harder to ignore and strained our relationship, but still I shrugged off mood swings and mishaps for too long. I ignored erratic behavior that wasn't at all in keeping with his nature.

Why didn't I insist sooner that we investigate the reasons Geoff was suffering so many falls—especially on those occasions when his injuries resulted in a trip to an emergency room? I should have, but I was more concerned in dealing with the immediate situation than the cause of it. Denial was another factor. It was preferable to fault a cracked sidewalk than consider the possibility Geoff might be developing a mobility issue. Had Geoff been examined earlier, we could have coped better with the mood swings and erratic behavior. It would have eased strains in our marital life. I would have been more vigilant, sparing Geoff so many unnecessary injuries.

If I could tap my earlier self on the shoulder and whisper in her ear, I'd tell her: *If you see something, say something.*

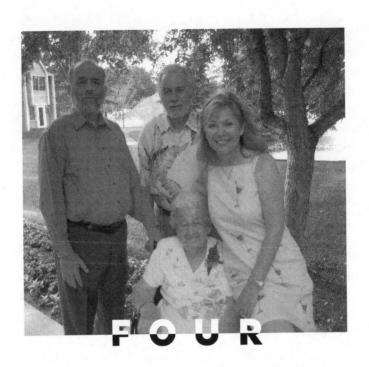

F O U R

"NO REGRETS"

Geoff and I flew together from Heathrow to New York's JFK airport. While he continued on to Los Angeles, where our friend Harry picked him up at the airport, I caught a flight to Minneapolis. As much as I urged him to come to Minneapolis with me, Geoff insisted he should return to Los Angeles to deal with bills and "hold down the fort."

My brother Orlyn met me at the airport in Minneapolis and took me directly to the hospital. My mother was sitting up in bed, looking surprisingly well and in full command. "Now, don't cry," she said. "I've decided." I gave her a hug and held her hand, somehow managing not to cry, which I knew would upset her.

But later, when her oncologist and a social worker spoke with my two brothers, their wives and me in a private conference room, none of us could hold back the tears. Her cancer had spread. My mother had chosen palliative care rather than an aggressive chemo treatment that might prolong her life for several months, at most. She made it clear that she preferred having a few comfortable weeks or months to put her life in order and say goodbye.

"There's no point in going through all that business. I've made my peace. I want to enjoy my life and keep my hair until it's over."

She also wanted to remain at home, and asked me to stay and care for her. That had been my plan as soon as I understood my mother's condition. I called Geoff and suggested that as soon as he'd taken care of mail and household matters in California he could join me in Minneapolis. My younger brother, David, and his wife, Kari, who lived in a spacious home on a lake near my mother's senior living residence, had invited Geoff to stay in their guest room. I would sleep on the couch in my mother's one-bedroom apartment.

"Let's give it a few days and see how things go," Geoff said. "You could be there for a while."

I agreed, yet I was concerned about Geoff staying alone while I was in Minneapolis, particularly as his head wound was still tender and healing. I called a couple of close friends and asked them to keep in touch with him, perhaps inviting him for a meal so he wouldn't be too lonely. Tim and David, who had married in our garden the year before, immediately dropped by the house to take Geoff for dinner.

Meanwhile, my mother was alert and looked much the same as when I'd last visited. She was taking various medications and had agreed to a form of palliative chemo treatment that would make her more comfortable. Otherwise her appetite was good and she was eager to watch her beloved Twins play ball. She was in such good spirits those first few days home from the hospital that I imagined she would be around throughout the entire baseball season, long beyond the six-weeks-to-three-months expiry date she'd been given. We very quickly fell into a routine. At first, she was able to bathe and dress herself, even make her own bed. I would organize her medications, prepare breakfast and then do whatever she directed me to do until my aunt joined her to watch *The Young and the Restless*. That was my chance to catch up on emails and make business calls.

Most of my time was spent following my mother's lead, assisting her with whatever she wanted to do. She had a surprising amount of energy. We went through her cedar chest, donated her books to the library, found a replacement for her on the altar guild and, as she said, "tidied up."

Her driver's license was due for renewal. "I don't s'pose I'll be driving much anymore," she said, "but I want to see if I can pass the test." She did. After her death, I framed her driver's license (good until June 2012) and put it on my desk.

We also visited my younger sister, who is profoundly mentally retarded as a result of an Rh-negative blood factor left untreated at birth. Sandra, who is unable to speak and has no cognitive ability, is well cared for in a group home where she's lived for many years. There are signs she recognizes us, and she occasionally smiles and returns a hug. That day, my sister seemed unusually receptive. My mother held her hand, fed her bits of chocolate we'd brought and hugged her goodbye. On our way home, my mother said, "You'll look after her, won't you?" I assured her I would. I'd long ago signed guardianship papers for my sister in the event of my mother's death.

My father had died at age ninety. As close and loving as my parents had been during their fifty-four years of marriage, my mother claimed that the years she'd lived on her own were some of the most secure and satisfying times of her life. She'd been born during the First World War, graduated from school during the Great Depression, married, borne children and lived as a farm wife during the Second World War. Immediately after the armistice was signed, our family was on the first passenger ship to war-torn Norway, where we lived on my father's farm for a year. We moved back to live in Minnesota only because of Sandra's health condition.

Life had not been easy, but my parents had created a warm, enriching family life that revolved around school events, church activities and cultural pursuits within the Norwegian-American community. They danced with a Norwegian folk dance group, did amateur theatrics and enjoyed a wide circle of friends. In her final weeks, Mother sat in front of her computer using Skype to get in touch with family in Norway and old friends living in distant places.

I wanted to make our days together fun and light-hearted, yet it was hard. She needed me and wanted me with her, but my presence got on her nerves. She couldn't bear having me constantly at hand, doing things for her that she wanted to do for herself, in her own way. She loved her solitude and also craved companionship, but it was hard to know just when to fulfill each of those desires. Our love for each other, and our patience, was sorely tested. She was particular and exacting about everything from watering plants to doing laundry and peeling potatoes. Nothing escaped her attention to detail. If she was displeased, she did not keep it a secret.

We had lots of good times together going for drives and stopping for malts and ice cream sundaes. On days when she had chemo, I'd take her for pancake breakfasts before her session because I knew she wouldn't want to eat afterward. Other days, after I'd helped her go through drawers, closets and cabinets, writing names on adhesive strips to identify items that were meant for someone special, I'd take my mother and aunt for lunch somewhere. Most afternoons, someone would drop by to see her. I'd set out coffee and cake and then sit in the garden with my laptop to give my mother some privacy with her visitors. I cooked dinner most evenings, with my aunt, brothers and other family members dropping by to visit.

If the Twins were playing, I would walk in the darkening twilight talking to Geoff on my cell phone. That's when I would cry and pour out my frustration.

"It's hard. She's difficult. Everything I do is wrong. She glares at me, ridicules me in front of guests. The oatmeal isn't right. I'm not fast enough. Then I'm rushing her. She pounds her fist on the table if I don't pour exactly the right amount of prune juice into her glass. I just can't please her!"

In his gentle way, Geoff would say, "No, you can't, so just roll with it. Stop looking for approval. She doesn't have time for that now. All you can hope for is not to have any regrets."

Afterward I'd sit on the warm, moonlit patio, swatting mosquitoes while my mother sat inside on her recliner, a Twins game playing on television. She'd watch in rapt stillness, a halo of lamplight shining on her perfectly coiffed white hair, a half-empty bowl of ice cream in her lap—then she'd suddenly bounce up and down, clapping her hands as a player scored a home run. I'd smile; sometimes cry. I was already missing her.

She'd look up, see me and say, "What are you doing out there? You can't still be talking to Geoff, for heaven's sake! Is something wrong with him?"

"No, no, he's fine."

"He should be here. Why isn't he here? There must be something wrong between you two."

Welcome to the soap opera world my mother and aunt inhabited. Neither could comprehend any reason why my husband—in my aunt's words, "retired and not doing anything, anyway"—wouldn't rather be with me "unless he's up to something."

I suspected my mother, an otherwise compassionate and loving soul, harbored the same sentiments. She had to be the center of *everyone's* universe, inhabiting a soap opera world of her own creation, fretting and manipulating in her role as family matriarch. It made me nuts. *Completely nuts.* I hated the drama and intrigue, the constant reading between the lines. She brooded when people (generally family members) didn't show up when she expected them for coffee or supper, although no invitation had been extended, no plan had been put in place, no phone call made—but "they should have known!" It became my personal mission to stamp out mental telepathy as the communication tool of choice in our family. I picked up the telephone, made sure everyone knew what was going on, and kept a daily schedule.

No regrets! No hurt feelings! Is such a thing achievable in any family?

But as much as we could grate on each other's nerves, I also took such overwhelming pride in her achievements. My mother had turned a menial job in a school lunchroom into a long and gratifying career in food services. Aware of every moment of my mother's declining health, I tried my very best to avoid regrets I'd carry with me the rest of my life. Her ninety-third birthday loomed, and I was in charge of organizing her party for the family in the garden atrium of her building. She knew what she wanted: chicken salad, fruit salad, walnut-banana bread, cloverleaf rolls, white wine and cake with coffee.

My mother also wanted to make her own *kransekake*, an elaborate Norwegian wedding cake made from hand-ground blanched almonds, egg whites and confectioner's sugar. I've made *kransekake* myself, a labor-intensive undertaking requiring approximately fifteen hand-rolled circles of almond dough baked in special tins. But I was thrilled to have a chance to make a *kransekake* under my mother's tutelage. She was, after all, the master *kransekake* baker in the Twin Cities.

Lacking the strength to do it herself, she sat on a stool watching as I hand-grated two pounds of blanched almonds, a small handful at a time, whisked egg whites by hand, sifted confectioner's sugar and then rolled the dough with my fingers to an exact nickel-size diameter. We managed this without bloodshed. The *kransekake* was perfection.

I arranged for Geoff to arrive the day before my mother's birthday. I picked him up at the airport and wrapped my arms around him, so grateful to see him again after nearly a month apart. "She's much weaker," I told him. "Still mean."

He laughed. I cried. "I love her. I'm already missing her. It's so *hard*."

"It's her journey," he reminded me. "Her death. Just be there for her."

Mother's birthday party was just as she wanted it. Her sister and brother, children, grandchildren, nephews, nieces and several close friends attended. We took family photographs in every conceivable combination. In the late afternoon I served coffee and cake. After Mother blew out ninety-three candles, she stood and spoke simply, her voice wavering only slightly as she acknowledged her end was near. How grateful she was, she said, that she could enjoy this occasion with the special people she loved most.

As I listened to her words, I appreciated her wisdom in choosing not to pursue all the aggressive treatments available to her. She was clearheaded, not foggy with medication. She had made her peace and wasn't clinging to last-minute reprieves. She looked lovely, her thick white hair styled perfectly. I'd taken her to the hairdresser and treated her to a spa manicure. She'd put on a pretty dress and her favorite pin and earrings. It was all just as she wanted it.

What she didn't want was for me to return to Los Angeles with Geoff. But I had to go back, at least for a few days. However much I'd been able to accomplish on my laptop, there were business matters I couldn't put off any longer. My mother appeared stable and in good spirits. She could live for many weeks, even months. However, there was no one to stay with her. My aunt was too frail to assist her. There were no family members available to give her the round-the-clock care she required.

My brothers and I looked into finding a facility where she would be well cared for and comfortable while I was gone. My mother was familiar with many of them because she'd seen friends "relegated" to them. She even accompanied us on a few exploratory visits to new places, but she wasn't happy about it. It angered her that with so little time left to her she couldn't remain at home. In hindsight, I wish we'd somehow convinced her to have nursing-care shifts in her own apartment, something she'd also rejected.

In the end, I packed up some framed photos, clothing, a few plants and a bouquet of flowers and moved her into what resembled a master suite in a Ritz-Carlton. This brand-new, very plush facility had been built on farmland near a creek where my mother, as our Brownie leader, had taken the troop on hikes and picnics. But the familiar view of cattails and willow trees on the shores of old Bassett's Creek didn't move her. Before I caught my flight, my mother, brothers and I all had lunch together in the spacious dining room. Mother picked at her food, suspicious of the herbs and raspberry vinaigrette. She glared disdainfully at the colorful nasturtiums garnishing her salad and flicked them off the plate with her butter knife. Then I left her, sitting on her plumped-up bed with the fancy brocade coverlet and tasseled pillows, looking forlorn.

"I'll only be gone a week," I assured her, my heart breaking at her obvious misery.

In fact, I was gone only four days. My mother was taken to hospital and I flew back as soon as I could get a flight. But during those four days in Los Angeles, it was clear to me that Geoff had struggled living by himself. Candelaria, our once-a-week housekeeper, had worked for Geoff for thirty-five years. She'd done an excellent job of maintaining order, but there were unmistakable signs that all was not well. Things were broken or left askew, containers were missing lids, drawers weren't closed, mail was stacked unopened and the suitcase he'd traveled with throughout Europe was still packed. Tim and David, who had taken him to dinner a couple of times, called to tell me he seemed "wobbly" and had trouble getting into their car. Gil and Miranda, close friends who had stopped by the house for a visit, said he appeared "a bit lost, distracted." I knew he'd been falling and bumping into things because I could see his bruises. I worried about the head injury he'd suffered in Italy, concerned there had been more damage than just a scalp wound. I hated leaving him alone again, but he refused to come with me.

Shortly after I returned to Minneapolis, my mother was put in hospice care. I spent every day with her, trying to make up for my absence. She was resentful that I'd left; her chilly reception let me know she felt betrayed and abandoned. It wasn't what she'd wanted.

Geoff warned me that she'd passed into a different phase, was pulling away. "Don't hold it against her," he said. "It's natural and she can't help it." He also told me I shouldn't take brusqueness or hurtful comments personally. But I did.

I knew Geoff was speaking from his own experience caring for his first wife, Barbara, during her twelve-year decline from MS. While Geoff ran the magazine, a caregiver had looked after Barbara during the day. But Geoff had looked after her by himself from evening to the following morning and throughout entire weekends. Still, as devoted and loving as he was, he regretted his own shortcomings.

"No matter what, there are regrets. It's unavoidable, but you try. Whatever you do, it's not going to be enough. There are times when you slip up, speak harshly, get irritable, and those are the times you remember afterward."

My mother passed away surrounded by family, a little over two months after her diagnosis. My brothers and I held her hands, remaining with her until her end.

Later, I returned to her apartment to choose clothing to bring to the mortuary, selecting a flattering navy blue suit Geoff had bought for her. Then I fell back onto her bed, sobbing, my arms and legs wheeling back and forth as though I were making snow angels on the coverlet. I breathed in her familiar scent on the pillows and cried hard. She'd been the precious anchor, the cornerstone of my life for sixty-some years. How could there be anything between us left unsaid, not done? But there were. Regrets? Of course!

Then I began recalling odd, fleeting, personal moments of connection... such as waking as a child and catching my mother late at night in the semi-dark of the farm kitchen, stitching a scrap of white satin. She'd looked up, caught my eye and tucked the satin between her knees. Weeks later, on Christmas Eve, after I opened my gift and found a storybook doll wearing an elegant hand-stitched satin wedding gown, I looked up and caught that look from her again. We may have been living in near poverty at the time, but my mother had managed to fulfill a little girl's dream with a homemade doll that was the most precious Christmas gift I've ever received. That's what I wanted to remember.

My mother's time of dying had initiated an intense, painfully personal journey between us that left me feeling raw and vulnerable. I'd wanted to be loving and patient throughout, but taking care of my mother had set off a role reversal neither of us was equipped to handle. Her loss of privacy and self-reliance had been deeply disturbing to a once strong, independent person.

As much as she'd needed me, she hadn't been prepared to relinquish her authority and dignity. I'd wanted my mom; she'd needed her daughter to assume an unexpected new role. I'd known her disease was terminal, but I hadn't fully taken into account the significance of the journey she'd begun. I hadn't accepted that her pulling away from me was as much a necessary part of her transition as my own pulling away to leave the family nest had once been for me.

Nor had I fully appreciated the effect her disease and medications had had on her demeanor. I took the harshness and irritability personally, despite Geoff's admonition at the time: *Remember, this is her journey. Just be there for her.* Although I took his words to heart at the time, I still harbored regret for the inevitable moments

of impatience and harshness when circumstances overwhelmed me.

And they would again, all too soon, when I was
caring for Geoff.

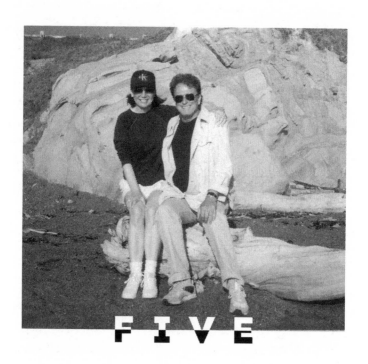

F I V E

"INDIAN SUMMER"

We had spent such a lot of time apart during my mother's illness that once Geoff and I were together again in Los Angeles, I was able to see him with fresh eyes—and I was concerned. Gestures that had once seemed idiosyncratic—such as the way he fumblingly adjusted his eyeglasses or awkwardly used only one hand to do the job of two—now struck me as odd behavior. Sitting with him at dinner, I found myself pressing my thumb against the base of a stemmed glass so that when he reached for it he couldn't tip it over.

I'd hoped the time apart would ease the tension that had been building up between us. It wasn't so much that we were bickering, but more that we were trying so hard not to do anything that would lead to an argument or hurt feelings. I made a point of not commenting in any way if Geoff tripped, stumbled or tipped something over. He hated being seen as clumsy or awkward, and avoided any situation that required dexterity.

Yet he would somehow manage to hurt himself doing the most ordinary task. Because he favored one hand, he would inevitably drop dishes, newspapers, cartons of milk, or injure himself lifting the lid on a rubbish bin. He was simply not capable of holding the lid up with one hand and using the other to toss in a sack of garbage. If he broke something, he became sullen. He didn't apologize. He didn't offer to clean up.

When Geoff retired from *Los Angeles* magazine, we'd joked that I would have to take over as "staff." In fact, "staff" became his funny nickname for me. Adding paper to the copy machine or wrapping a package were tasks he could not handle because of his growing difficulty coordinating two hands. He'd try to fill ice cube trays in the old refrigerator in the garage where we kept beer, wine, bottled water and juices. Hours later I would find pools of water on the garage floor and the ice cube trays in the freezer compartment barely filled.

When we gave dinner parties, it was Geoff's job to "set the scene." While I worked in the kitchen, he lit candles, chose music, filled the wine bucket with ice and set glasses on the bar. But on a couple of occasions I found him struggling to open bottles of white wine hours before dinner. Once, I stopped him from opening a bottle of champagne more than an hour before guests were to arrive.

"Stop! Why are you doing that?"

"I don't want to be stuck opening bottles when everyone's watching me."

"But it's too early."

"Then do it yourself."

So I did—and also took on the job of lighting the gas logs in the fireplace when it became dangerously apparent that Geoff could no longer do it. One evening I smelled gas and found Geoff sitting on the living room couch trying to reach the gas peg while struggling to click the fire starter.

"You could have blown us up!"

"I've been doing this for forty years," he shouted. "If you don't like the way I do it—"

"Use two hands! You can't do this without getting on your knees and turning the gas on with one hand and lighting the logs with the other."

"So you do it!"

Doing everything came at a price. The more I took on, the less confident Geoff became. If he was slow to do something, I stepped in and then bore the brunt of his frustration. "You just have to show me up, don't you?"

Geoff, who had always been a warm, gracious host, deft with conversation and full of good stories, had begun to fall silent once the meal was served. He'd prop his elbow on the table, lean awkwardly over his plate and use only one hand to eat. He handled a soupspoon like a shovel and couldn't manage to hold a fork to eat salad. Most annoying, his eyelids would droop and he looked bored or appeared to be falling asleep while dining. I'd nudge him awake and he'd look at me in surprise, as though unaware he'd been eating with his eyes closed.

I'd continually remind Geoff not to clutch his wine glass but set it on the table; to use both his fork and knife; to take smaller bites so he wouldn't choke; and to *please, please* cover his mouth when he coughed. I sounded like the dreaded hall monitor, or the nanny from hell. Geoff was sick of hearing "a laundry list of complaints." Sometimes we argued; often we rode home in silence after an evening out. I could not understand how he could have become so oblivious and ill-mannered, and he wondered why I'd stopped loving him.

"You never used to complain," he'd say.

True. No matter how hard I tried not to, I'd begun to complain a lot. So I saved my complaints for important things, such as, "Please shower and get dressed so we can leave on time!"

Then, as we were walking out the door, I'd notice he wasn't wearing socks, or had forgotten his belt. My husband, who had always cared about his appearance, was no longer willing to wear certain shoes, pants or shirts. We struggled and argued over the most mundane things.

It wasn't until one evening late that summer, when we were getting dressed for a black-tie event, that I realized how difficult it was for him to get dressed. I ended up helping him with everything, including his socks and shoes. I teased him about needing a butler and gave him a kiss, hoping our evening wouldn't be spoiled.

Life was becoming a lot less fun. Too often I'd offer help when he didn't want it, which annoyed him. Worse, I failed to notice when he did need help. Frustrated, he'd give up and we'd suffer the consequences.

"Why didn't you just ask me to put your belt through the loops?"

"I didn't want to bother you."

At the least sign of exasperation from either of us, tempers flared and we ended up saying hurtful things neither of us meant.

"Leave me alone! You don't love me anymore. Divorce me!"

"I don't want a divorce. I just want you to put on a clean shirt."

We loved each other, and our marriage would not come to an end over table manners and wardrobe issues. But anger, frustration, resentment and hurtful words were taking a terrible toll. I made every sort of adjustment and concession to avoid trouble, which meant we no longer talked about or did some of the things we'd once enjoyed together.

The problems we were dealing with escalated so quickly that by the late summer of 2007 I was convinced that some medical condition was causing these changes. I didn't think it was the onset of Alzheimer's, because he wasn't particularly forgetful. He followed the stock market as avidly as ever and handled our finances well. He loved language and was skillful with words, although his handwriting was no longer as legible. Letters and numbers were ill formed and cramped. Occasionally there was a bit of inappropriate behavior, but it seemed to have more to do with a physical struggle than a mental disconnect. I traced the difficulties back to the head injury in Italy, but Geoff insisted the wound had healed and refused to see a doctor.

One afternoon I glanced out the window, horrified to see Geoff on the street in bare feet, half dressed, trying to open our mailbox. He was tugging at the key with one hand and, when the latch suddenly opened, almost fell backward into the street. Then he reached into the box and grabbed the mail with one hand, dropping half of it on the pavement.

I flew down the stairs and raced outside, furious with him. I picked up the mail, grabbed the key, slammed the box closed and herded Geoff back inside. He couldn't understand why I was so upset that he'd walked out of the house and onto a public street wearing nothing more than Fruit of the Looms and a skimpy robe flapping open. But then it occurred to me that he'd become so frustrated trying to get dressed that he'd just given up.

All he wanted to do was get the mail, another routine task that had become difficult for him. He had to keep his balance while working the key in the lock, opening the latch and juggling an armload of mail, all using one hand. From then on it was my job to get the mail in the afternoon and fetch the newspapers in the morning.

Geoff and I belonged to a health club that we regularly attended together. While I worked out, Geoff would occupy a treadmill at "stroll" speed and watch reruns of *The Rockford Files*. One evening he came out of the men's changing room half-dressed because he couldn't get his pants buttoned and zipped. He stood leaning against the wall in the reception area, his pants hanging on his hips, waiting for me to come out of the women's locker room to help him. I was appalled that he was so oblivious to the people around him. I hustled him into a nearby exercise room and helped him get dressed.

"You have to remember who you are, and where you are . . . you have to be more aware, Geoff."

He started laughing. "Are you aware you have your hands on my crotch?"

I looked around the mirrored room and realized everyone passing by could see me on my knees struggling with his zipper. I laughed along with him.

More worrying were the mobility and balance problems that were causing frequent falls and injuries. One night, after a dinner party in the upper garden, Geoff fell while trying to put the cover back on the grill. I was in the kitchen washing up and assumed Geoff was clearing the bar area and listening to a jazz CD. It had long been our custom, once guests left and the cleaning up was done, to sit at the candlelit table having a last glass of wine and listening to music.

When I finished washing up, I went to the upper garden carrying two glasses of wine. But as I made my way up the steps, I saw trails of blood and bloody footprints. I looked around, calling his name, then raced across the little bridge connecting the garden to our bedroom. There were splotches of blood everywhere on the carpet and doorway.

Geoff was in the bathroom, running water in the sink. As soon as he saw me, he said, "I'm sorry I made a mess. I was hoping to clean it up." His cheek, knees, hands and arms were bloody from cuts and scrapes.

"But you should have called me!"

"I don't need you to get mad at me."

"I'm not mad. You're hurt. I could have helped you."

"I didn't want to bother you."

He'd lost a lot of blood and I was afraid he might go into shock. I told him I was going to call the paramedics. He wouldn't allow it. I asked if he'd bumped his head. He said he hadn't. I helped him into a chair so I could check his injuries and clean him up.

"What happened? Do you remember how you fell?"

"I tripped . . . had trouble getting up."

I remembered seeing an overturned patio chair and realized he must have used it while struggling to get back on his feet. Every conceivable scenario flashed before my eyes—he could have blacked out, fallen in the pool, slipped on the stone steps and broken bones. He was trembling, and I was certain the "what ifs" were on his mind, too.

After cleaning him up, I determined that the cuts and scrapes were superficial, but I was still concerned he might have other injuries I wasn't aware of. I suggested we sit on the couch for a while and calm ourselves. He still seemed shaky and I wanted to make sure he wasn't feeling dizzy or ill before I helped him to bed. We held hands and talked, neither of us mentioning concerns about Geoff's mobility problems and frequent falls.

Oddly enough, we started talking about traveling again, perhaps out of an unconscious desire to distance ourselves from more immediate concerns. In any case, a frivolous late-night chat led to plans for a visit to the Greek Isles.

We'd taken a very enjoyable Baltic cruise to St. Petersburg with the Oceania line. The ship was able to dock at the English Embankment, almost directly in front of the Hermitage Museum, instead of a terminal some distance from the city, which was only one of the advantages of being on a smaller ship. I saw that the line was offering special rates on a Mediterranean cruise in late October that would take us from Venice to Istanbul. On impulse, I signed up. It would give us something to look forward to and perhaps take our minds off a sad and difficult summer.

In the meantime, I did rewrites on a novel. I was also preparing the final draft of my article on Birgit Nilsson, "The Star and the Stalker," to send to *Opera News*. I was in my office finishing up the feature piece when the doorbell rang. A woman with a clipboard was standing on the front steps. She identified herself as an agent with our insurance company and said she had scheduled an appointment with Geoff. He hadn't mentioned the meeting to me.

On the way up to Geoff's office, I asked her if there was a problem. "There was an incident we need to talk about. He didn't tell you?"

"No. Is it serious?" By that time we were in Geoff's office and I asked him, "What's this about?"

"Somebody filed a complaint, that's all. I didn't want to bother you."

That phrase again! "Okay, do you mind if I sit in?"

Geoff rolled his eyes. "I thought you had a deadline."

"I do. I'm wrapping it up." The agent gave each of us her card and took a seat. "Please start without me," I told her. "I'll be back as soon as I can."

By the time I returned, the agent had spread grainy pictures and photocopies of various documents on Geoff's desk. "What happened? When was this?" I asked.

"Last June. You were in Minneapolis with your mother. I didn't want to upset you. In fact, nothing much happened."

The "nothing much happened" incident had been designated a felony hit-and-run. Geoff was stopped at a traffic light at the bottom of a freeway exit ramp. As the light changed, a young woman jogger darted across traffic. Geoff had already released his brake and was moving forward. The jogger ran into his car and, bracing her hands against the hood, leaped back. From the POV of an off-duty school bus driver several cars back on the exit ramp, it appeared that Geoff's car had struck the woman and continued into the intersection without stopping.

Geoff said he didn't feel an impact but knew something had happened. He looked for a place to pull over, and then saw the woman continuing her jog. He drove several more blocks, turned around and found a parking place. He eventually spoke with the woman, who told him she wasn't injured.

Another witness saw Geoff speaking with her. However, the bus driver had already taken down Geoff's license plate number and reported the incident. Furthermore, when the young jogger got home and told her boyfriend about the close call, he insisted on taking her to an emergency room.

Almost two months after the incident, Geoff was charged with felony hit-and-run. He'd made every poor choice imaginable, but I believed his version of the events. I knew he was a careful driver, who didn't "jackrabbit" when traffic lights changed. He had an unblemished driving record and had returned to check on the jogger. But I also believed the jogger, who noted that Geoff seemed "befuddled" and "not in control." Those descriptions appeared several times in various depositions, including the statement of the bus driver. I wondered if Geoff's "tunnel vision" had come into play; he'd developed a habit of not looking to his right or left.

Before Geoff's court appearance, we met with an attorney. With evidence that Geoff had returned to speak with the jogger and hospital records indicating she had no injuries that required treatment, the charge was reduced to a misdemeanor.

We dressed up for the court appearance, Geoff in suit and tie and me in a dark suit and pumps. Our exotic apparel drew stares from defendants dressed in shorts and flip-flops, but I thought it was important for Geoff to look like someone substantial and responsible—at the very least, someone capable of knotting a necktie. In fact, I had to help him with both the necktie and cufflinks. But when he approached the bench with the attorney, he shuffled, appeared hesitant and, to my eyes, looked *befuddled*. I was not surprised when his driver's license was suspended. He was also fined and assigned community service.

Afterward, while I raced around from one department to another, paying the fine and gathering documents, Geoff stood in line waiting to be assigned community service. He was the only man wearing a suit—also, the only one having difficulty standing on his feet.

When I rejoined him, I saw that Geoff had been pushed ahead in the line. Several of the other men looked at me and shook their heads. "Your man," one said to me in broken English, "he no stand. He fall down. You tell." He waggled his thumb at the cubicles where clerks were assigning road maintenance work.

By this time, Geoff, who admitted he'd fallen onto the marble floor and been lifted back on his feet by the other men in line, was so weak he had to sit on a bench. I took his place in the queue.

Clearly Geoff would not be assigned a luminescent orange vest and ordered to pick up trash along the Ventura Freeway. Instead, he was consigned to an HIV/AIDS food distribution center. The following Monday morning, I packed a lunch and drove him to a facility deep in the San Fernando Valley, where he was put to work sorting food donations from eight o'clock in the morning until four o'clock in the afternoon. I gave him a kiss goodbye and he waved me off. I knew he didn't want me watching him struggle to unpack a crate of lettuce.

I slipped back into the warehouse office and left my card. "If anything happens to him, please call me." I also offered to stay and help, but was turned away. By the time I returned in the afternoon, Geoff had been reassigned to the front desk, filling brown paper bags with assorted foodstuffs. He was scowling and clearly frustrated that he couldn't open bags without ripping them, nor could he coordinate his hands to pick up cans and jars. One of the clients waiting in line complained loudly that Geoff was too slow and inefficient.

When we got in the car, Geoff was glum. "They gave me a two-hour lunch break," he said. "Could I have an extra sandwich tomorrow?"

Our goal was to finish the community service requirement before our cruise. It gave us a goal, something to look forward to. Aside from time off for a doctor's appointment, Geoff worked six to eight hours a day, five days a week, often just serving as a "greeter," watching clients sign in at the door. Eventually, he was reassigned to various grocery store collection sites. One Saturday, Geoff sat at a table outside a Gelson's store in Silver Lake, chatting with people donating groceries. He felt he'd finally found his calling. He was exuberant on our drive home, telling me about some of the people he'd met.

"You know, most of the people dropping off groceries have AIDS themselves," he marveled. "And someone bought me coffee." He also instructed me to buy a bag of groceries to donate. Then he wept.

Geoff was genuinely touched by the experience, but he'd begun to weep spontaneously with little control of his emotions. Listening to music moved him deeply and often brought on tears. When he quoted poetry or read aloud a touching passage from a book, tears filled his eyes. He was especially susceptible to song lyrics by Johnny Mercer and Cole Porter. Whatever caused him to weep, these brief, tearful moments seemed genuine and heartfelt—but they were also becoming all too frequent.

I was concerned enough about Geoff's emotional state, erratic behavior and mobility problems that I pressured him into seeing his primary care physician. Once we were in the waiting room, I persuaded Geoff to let me speak with the doctor myself. I knew that on his own, Geoff would have an amiable chat without ever mentioning the problems he was having. He reluctantly permitted me to accompany him into the examining room, but warned me not to "rattle off a laundry list of complaints about me." As tactfully as I could, I prompted Geoff to mention his recent falls and the circumstances of the traffic misdemeanor.

Meanwhile, I saw the doctor observe some of the symptoms I had noticed. Geoff no longer looked at the person he was talking to. He couldn't stand on one foot. He couldn't coordinate his hands, and one hand made involuntary waving movements. An obvious initial diagnosis was some form of Parkinson's, although Geoff had no tremors or other outward signs of the disease. The doctor sent Geoff for an MRI and other tests, none of which revealed strokes, inner ear problems, or anything relating to the head injury in Italy.

Geoff was relieved. I was anxious. I knew something was wrong. I suspected he did not tell me about falls when I wasn't around unless I happened to notice that he had skinned knees, bruised legs, cuts or stiff joints. I was secretly glad his driver's license had been suspended. Months before the accident, I'd been aware he was no longer the skilled driver he'd once been. He would drive too slowly, stop abruptly and appear to be driving on what I began calling "remote control."

If he listened to KJAZZ on the radio, he would drive as though tapping his foot in time to the music, or slow up for no reason. He never seemed to look to the left or right. But now, prevented from driving, he was entirely dependent on me, and that created even more tension. I sympathized with his desire not to let anyone know he'd lost his license. I concocted excuses that would explain why I was dropping him off for lunch with one of his pals and picking him up afterward. He would come with me on errands, which he enjoyed, and I would leave him at a newsstand while I did my shopping. One of Geoff's most enjoyable pastimes was spending an hour or so perusing magazine racks, a sort of busman's holiday. Still, there was no way around the fact that Geoff was now tied to me, and he resented his lack of freedom. We were experiencing the sorts of tensions I'd had with my mother. He needed me, wanted me on call, but resented having to rely on me. It was not fun.

We were both looking forward to the cruise. With Geoff's community service behind us, we prepared for our trip. To break up the long direct flight to Venice, we planned to spend a week in New York. Geoff was thrilled. He'd be able to get out of the apartment and walk around town by himself. Before leaving on our trip, I invested in sturdy rubber-soled walking shoes and Dockers with elastic waistbands. I also packed sweaters and pullover shirts so he could more easily dress himself. He still preferred wearing blue jeans and safari jackets most of the time, and I was quick to give him a hand with zippers and buttons.

But more importantly, Geoff only had the impression of being alone. I arranged to accompany him almost everywhere. We went to Birdland together and I spent whole days exploring his favorite haunts with him. I was happy to let him take charge in planning our outings and he seemed happy (relieved?) to have my company.

The cruise was a tonic. Because our ship was relatively small, not one of the behemoths with thousands of passengers, we could take our time disembarking. When most of the other passengers had left, we made our way onto the dock, strolling leisurely and stopping in a café when Geoff tired. To my surprise, he was able to walk for several hours in Taormina and Amalfi and we didn't return to our ship until late afternoon.

Geoff appeared revitalized and had no problems negotiating steep climbs and the narrow passages we encountered while visiting the hilltop village of Santo-rini or the winding streets of Rhodes, where we bought each other leather jackets. We explored the Parthenon in Athens, Greece, and the ancient ruins in Kusadasi, Turkey, without mishap or a single stumble. We spent two days in Istanbul, visiting the markets, walking eve-rywhere. Aboard ship, Geoff had no difficulty navi-gating the decks and corridors of the ship by himself and enjoyed the solitude of sitting quietly in a deck chair.

Again, we broke the long flight with a week's stay in New York before returning to Los Angeles. On the way home, Geoff suggested we spend Christmas in New York and go to London for New Year's, another ambitious round of travel. We had plenty of airline miles and places to stay in both cities—the trip wouldn't be costly, so why not? I booked the tickets because Geoff seemed to thrive on all the travel and activity. He was happier than I had seen him in a long time. We were together constantly, walking everywhere—so perhaps the combination of exercise, companionship, stimulat-ing social life and activity provided all the therapy he needed.

Seeing signs of improvement made me wonder if I'd been imagining problems. Perhaps he'd had small, undetectable strokes and was recovering. His speech was no longer slurred. He laughed easily, told stories and engaged in conversation during dinner. There were no angry outbursts or periods of sullenness. Whatever the storm was, I began to think we'd weathered it and passed into calmer waters. Travel was the answer!

Still, I took nothing for granted. I was vigilant wher-ever we went, keeping a sharp eye out for any potential hazard that might cause him to slip, fall or injure himself. I instinctively took his arm when we walked or climbed stairs and gave him a hand when he sat down or stood up. We now routinely showered together, with Geoff holding on to faucets while I bathed him. When he insisted on taking the subway, I was on the lookout for elevators to avoid escalators, and kept a firm grip on his arm. We did not take buses.

Life was almost normal again. We entertained, had dinner with friends, went to theatre and concerts—and it became second nature for me to mask any awkward behavior on Geoff's part. When visiting friends, I made sure Geoff sat in a chair he could get out of again. On more than one occasion, under the guise of tasting something on Geoff's plate, I quickly cut up meat into bite-size pieces.

But on New Year's Eve, only an hour into a black-tie party in the home of friends in London, Geoff grew pale and became so unsteady that I made excuses and we left before the buffet dinner. He was upset he'd spoiled my evening, but I convinced him that the warm, crowded room had made me uncomfortable, too. I don't think I was even aware of how very watchful I was, nor of all the small adjustments and accommodations I made to keep him safe. I wanted us to be normal, to keep Geoff happy and comfortable. Since I was always holding his hand or gripping his arm, we must have looked like the most loving couple on the planet.

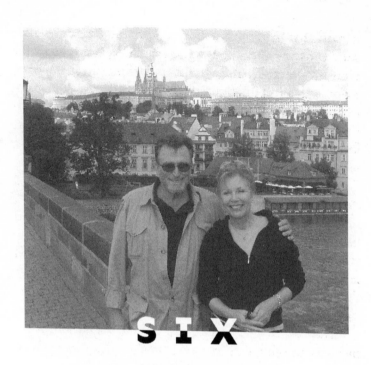

SIX

"DON'T WORRY 'BOUT ME"

Geoff and I were inseparable. I rarely left him alone at home, taking him with me everywhere I went. When we shopped for groceries, Geoff pushed the cart, which served as convenient support. One afternoon, I noticed a woman watching me as we were moving through the aisles. When I caught her eye, she looked away. I figured she probably recognized me as an actress, which turned out to be the case. Before reaching the checkout, Geoff said he was getting tired and wanted to wait for me in the car. I walked to the parking lot with him, helped him into the car and then returned to the store.

The woman, attractive and about my age, approached me in the checkout lane and said, "Excuse me, but I've seen you on television. I know who you are. I didn't mean to stare, but I understand what you're going through. Does he have Parkinson's?"

"No, nothing like that. He's fine."

"Sorry, I thought he might have what my husband has," she said. "I hope you don't mind the intrusion."

"Not at all, but I'm so sorry about your husband. I wish you the best."

"Thank you. You, too." She smiled, then added, "You know, you're very good with him. It's not easy."

The woman was pleasant and clearly meant well, but I wasn't prepared for her comments. In the parking lot I gripped the handle of the grocery cart, trying to control my emotions. I'd thought we were normal again, but other people, even strangers, could see something was wrong.

On the way home, Geoff told me he wanted to take a driving test so he could get his license back. I tried to stall him, but a few days later he called the DMV on his own and made an appointment. I drove him to the testing center, where he passed the written exam with a near perfect score. This wasn't surprising, since two of the most popular features Geoff introduced to *Los Angeles* magazine were the answers to the DMV driving test and a map of surface street shortcuts to avoid traffic.

Before Geoff took his road test, I drove him around

the surrounding streets so he could familiarize himself with the neighborhood. In the DMV parking lot I let him take the wheel to practice driving. My heart sank when I realized he was unable to maintain steady pressure on the gas pedal and had little control over his foot. He'd jerk to a stop or drive so slowly we were barely moving. I saw the bewildered look on his face and tried to encourage him. It was no surprise to either of us when he failed the driving test.

He wanted a second chance. A month later, after a full morning of intense practice in the DMV parking lot, Geoff passed the road test. Without comment, he handed me his car keys, and I drove us home. We arranged to sell his cherished convertible and have his name removed from our automobile insurance policy. Our premium had skyrocketed after his accident, but I'd paid it without comment. He'd wanted to prove he could pass the test and decide for himself when he should stop driving, just as my mother had.

For the first time that spring, I accompanied Geoff to the Monterey Jazz Festival, driving his favored route and stopping at the Cold Spring Tavern for lunch. He'd always enjoyed having this weekend to himself, strolling from one venue to the next, listening to his beloved "moldy fig" traditional jazz. I tried to make myself as scarce as possible. Once he was seated, I would leave him on his own. But he also enjoyed introducing me to his special haunts, a restaurant that served great crab cakes and a breakfast hangout where he could get buckwheat flapjacks with genuine maple syrup.

Back in Los Angeles, Geoff and I made an appointment with a neurologist recommended by a friend who had recently been diagnosed with Parkinson's disease. I helped Geoff fill out the new-patient forms, but he did not want me in the examining room with him.

"Let Dr. C figure out what's wrong with me instead of you coming up with all sorts of things," he said. "There's nothing wrong with my ears and I haven't had a stroke." I remained in the waiting room.

After his appointment, Geoff told me Dr. C wasn't sure what he had, but that it wasn't Parkinson's. He handed me a prescription for Sinemet, which we filled at the pharmacy on our way home. Back in my office, I looked up Sinemet on the Internet and saw that it was a brand name for carbidopa/levodopa, used in the treatment of Parkinson's disease. When I mentioned this to Geoff, he shrugged and said, "Yeah, I know. He just wanted to see if it would make any difference."

Geoff started taking the drug and we both looked for signs of improvement. For a while, we even imagined Sinemet had restored Geoff's ability to walk without weaving and wobbling, which emboldened us to make more travel plans. We set off for another extended trip to New York and London, where I had work and meetings lined up in both cities. In London, I'd been booked to do audio recordings over a period of several days. I tried to entice Geoff to go to the studio with me, but he preferred spending his time in the Cottage. He seemed so improved that I didn't worry about leaving him on his own.

The recording studio happened to be near the home of our close friends, Adrian and Jo-an, so we arranged to meet them for dinner when I finished my last day of work. Geoff still loved London buses and had begun riding them alone again, although I made him promise not to climb to the top level. I tried to persuade him to take a taxi to meet me, but he insisted on taking a bus. The route wasn't complicated, and he promised to sit on the lower level. I wrote out instructions, made sure his cell phone was working and told him I would wait at the bus stop in front of the studio so he would see me.

In the end, Geoff forgot both the instructions and the cell phone at home, took the wrong bus and went missing for three hours. By nine o'clock that evening, I was frantic. The friends we were supposed to meet for dinner drove the length of the bus route looking for him. Finally we returned to the Cottage and began calling area hospitals.

Nearly an hour later Geoff arrived home, feigning nonchalance and pretending not to understand our concern. But despite his bravado, it was clear to all of us that he was confused and shaken by his misadventure. Later, in bed, Geoff confessed he'd also forgotten to take his wallet. A sympathetic taxi driver had brought him home after Geoff described where he lived. The cabdriver had given him his card, and the following morning I mailed a check to cover the fare and a generous tip for his exceptional kindness.

The incident left us both subdued for days afterward. Geoff lost some of his trademark bonhomie, no longer able to ignore his diminishing abilities and increasing reliance on me. I felt guilty that I hadn't taken him with me to the studio, or insisted that he take a taxi instead of a bus. He wanted to remain in denial, but I didn't have that option. I had failed him by not being more alert in protecting him from situations I should have known he couldn't handle.

But staying with Geoff around the clock was not

an option, either. It wasn't possible or desirable for either of us. We needed our time apart. Engaging a paid companion/caregiver, which Geoff did not necessarily want or need, would have completely compromised his game of denial. The immediate solution for me was to eliminate any personal outings that weren't necessary and to make sure I didn't leave Geoff alone for too long.

I was willing to cut back but not to entirely stop working. The real strain was managing my professional appointments and obligations in those circumstances when I had little flexibility. Back in New York, I filmed a television commercial, attended some meetings at BookExpo and met with a producer interested in filming a documentary based on "The Star and the Stalker."

The arrangements I made for Geoff when I had to leave him alone weren't ideal. My meetings were hurried because I always had one eye on my watch. Filming on location was even more stressful because I had no control over when we would wrap the shoot. When I filmed a commercial on location in New Jersey, I relied on a friend to make lunch for Geoff and arranged for the doorman to check on him periodically.

Friends were accommodating, but I tried not to make it look like I was using them as "sitters" even when the more intuitive ones offered to serve that very purpose. Geoff was generally cheerful about my tight scheduling, but every move involved negotiation. He demanded to know *exactly* when I would return. I couldn't be late. If I thought I would be delayed, I'd call the doorman to relay the message because I couldn't risk calling Geoff. On several occasions he'd dropped the phone on the floor and was unable to pick it up. Alarmed when I heard a busy signal, I would panic and race home to find that he'd accidentally kicked the phone across the floor and couldn't reach it.

Fortunately our apartment was on the ground floor. I could leave the door unlatched and ask the doorman to look in on him occasionally. The arrangement gave me some peace of mind, but I still worried. There were also times when Geoff would stubbornly refuse to go along with what he called my "marching orders."

Late one afternoon, Geoff and I were sitting in the garden area of our New York apartment building, waiting for an old friend to join us for dinner at a nearby restaurant. I asked Geoff to remain in the garden while I went back into our apartment to get sweaters. The phone rang while I was inside and I was delayed several minutes. As I stepped out of the apartment with the sweaters, I saw Geoff slumped between the building manager and a doorman, his arms draped across their shoulders, his feet dragging on the marble floor. His face was cut and he was covered in shards of glass.

Instead of waiting in the garden for me to return, Geoff had tried to climb the flight of steep steps by himself. He'd tumbled backward down the stairs and struck his head on the door, smashing wood and glass panes. The marble floor was thick with shattered debris, including glittering wedges of broken glass and sharp sticks of wood—how had he survived? Yet even as I reached out to him with shaking hands, Geoff smiled and said, "Nothing to worry about. Didn't want to bother you."

I stared in exasperation, the sweater I'd brought for him slung across my arm. "Why couldn't you wait?" It was a useless question for which there was no answer.

The building manager wanted to call paramedics, but Geoff refused. "I'm fine," he said. "I fell slowly. Nothing broken. I don't want to go to the hospital."

We eased him onto a bench and I checked his injuries. I asked if he'd struck his head in the fall and he said he hadn't. The cuts and scrapes were superficial and he felt no tenderness when I touched the back of his head. By that time our friend had arrived in the lobby and Geoff insisted upon going into our apartment.

Paramedics should have been called. Why hadn't I insisted? But again, with Geoff joking and laughing, the moment of urgency passed. He seemed fine. While our friend sat talking with him, I hooked up the Hoover to vacuum glass shards from his hair and clothing. He thought it was funny and joked about being "hard-headed."

"You should have stayed in the garden and this wouldn't have happened," I scolded.

"I wanted to come in," he said pointedly. "If I want to do something, I'll do it. I don't need your permission."

I made dinner at home. My friend stayed until late in the evening, both of us alert to any changes in Geoff's condition. The building manager looked in on us several times. But Geoff didn't have a headache or nausea. His color was good and he showed no difficulty in his speech. He slept soundly that night. I didn't. I got out of bed, put on a robe and went to the lobby to take another look at the scene of the accident. The glass had been swept up, the broken panes covered with cardboard. I stared at the marble steps, picturing Geoff falling backward, his head crashing through the thick glass—and felt sick to my stomach.

The incident was a defining moment. It was clear to me there would no longer be a "normal" in our lives. I could not pretend that all I had to do was stay close to home and hold Geoff's hand to keep him safe. He wasn't "fine" by any stretch of the imagination. It was becoming clear to everyone. After that fall, the staff in the building treated us differently, with everyone alert to Geoff's balance problems. Trying to cover up Geoff's wobbliness or laughing off the spills and stumbles was no longer possible. I asked myself why I'd been so slow in acknowledging how serious Geoff's problems were, and the answer was clear: I was in my own state of denial. I didn't want to face it. I wanted none of it to happen, nothing to change.

But we had to deal with it. I persuaded Geoff to see a doctor in New York, who had been highly recommended as a specialist in Parkinson's disease. But the only appointment available was on an afternoon when I'd already scheduled a lunch meeting with a documentary film producer. Although the restaurant happened to be near the doctor's office, I told Geoff I would come back to the apartment to pick him up. He was adamant about taking a taxi alone to the doctor's office.

"There's no need to come back for me. What can happen?" he said. "It's twelve blocks! If you're going to baby me, I'm not going."

Again, we were embroiled in negotiation—over a taxi ride! In the end I agreed to his terms. I made sure he had money in the pocket of his safari jacket, gave the doorman the doctor's address and asked him to help Geoff get into a taxi. At the appointed time, I nervously waited for him on the street outside the doctor's office. He arrived only a few minutes late, but he was agitated and fearful. His face was tight, his eyes huge and anxious.

Climbing out of the cab, he mumbled, "It wasn't a good idea."

I didn't mention that it was *his* idea. I gave him a hug and took his shaking hand. Later, he confided that he couldn't stop himself from sliding off the seat onto the floor of the taxi. The driver had had to pull over, help him back up onto the seat and buckle him in.

We waited a few minutes in the reception room, which gave Geoff a chance to calm himself. Dr. B, elderly and urbane, was nearing retirement, as was his slightly daffy and delightful receptionist. Geoff was put at ease as soon as we entered the doctor's office, a cozy den with leather wing chairs.

The two men quickly bonded over their mutual love for jazz and swing-era big bands. It took me several minutes to realize the doctor was cleverly taking Geoff's medical history and evaluating his memory and cognitive skills by getting him to talk about music. Dr. B checked Geoff's reflexes and mobility, and seemed particularly interested in the fact that when Geoff fell, he fell backward—and that he had difficulty coordinating his hands.

"You don't have Parkinson's," he told Geoff, "but possibly a condition sometimes referred to as Parkinson-plus. There's no available medication for it, but keep taking the Sinemet for now." He administered a vitamin B shot, wrote a prescription for another medication to try, and told us he would arrange for Geoff to see a neurologist at New York-Presbyterian/Columbia University Medical Center the next time we were in New York.

"He may be doing some clinical trials. I'll give you a referral. There's also a fellow at the Mayo Clinic you might want to see. In the meantime, stay as physically and mentally active as you can."

We both took this as good news—which probably had much to do with the doctor's genial personality. I filled the prescription for the new medication and then discovered on the Internet that the drug Aricept was primarily prescribed for Alzheimer's patients. I was surprised the doctor thought the medication was necessary for Geoff, who had shown impressive knowledge and recall in their conversation together.

I did not tell Geoff what the medication was for, both to preserve his state of denial and to keep him from losing confidence in his mental state. Unfortunately, Geoff made the connection one afternoon when he saw a television commercial for the product. "So now I'm losing my marbles, too."

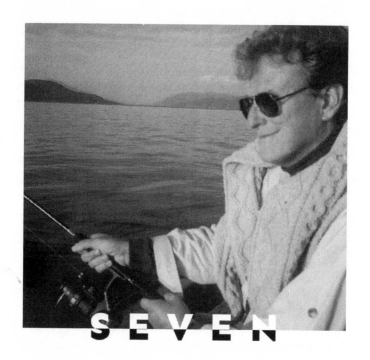

S E V E N

"THE MAN I LOVE"

Back in Los Angeles, I followed Dr. B's advice to keep Geoff physically and mentally active. We were both on the board of our homeowners' association, so I assisted Geoff in writing an article for the newsletter about film star Jacqueline Bisset, who lived in our neighborhood. It was easy to arrange a meeting, since she and I had once played sisters in a motion picture, and she'd also appeared on a cover of *Los Angeles* magazine. We met at her home and I took notes while Geoff interviewed her. Afterward, he dictated the article to me, a delightful piece that was the lead story in the newsletter.

I signed both of us up with the Plato Society, a program for seniors at UCLA that coordinated independent study groups on a wide variety of subjects. Our first topic was Women of the Left Bank, based on women literary figures in 1920s Paris. We would meet on Tuesday mornings for a full semester, each participant assigned to lead a weekly discussion on a particular topic. Geoff would make his presentation on Janet Flannery one week, and I would lead a discussion on Djuna Barnes another week. We crammed and prepared like crazy, having a wonderful time working together.

But with our good intentions and willingness to pursue new things, we also opened the door to the harsh reality of just how much Geoff's abilities had diminished. In a roomful of retired academics and accomplished professionals, most of them older than us, Geoff's difficulties speaking, reading and writing stood out—and this wasn't a sympathetic crowd. Signing up for Plato meant committing to rigorous study and preparation for intense, intellectually competitive discussions. Participants also adhered to two inviolate rules that pleased us: No talk about grandchildren or personal ailments.

As much as Geoff enjoyed the stimulating sessions, he was also made acutely aware of his shortcomings. We were among strangers who had never experienced Geoff's agile mind or his quick wit, and I was not in a position to surreptitiously cover for him. It was painful to feel him struggling to keep up when he'd once been so deft at debate. But I was gratified to notice a faint hush of expectancy when he did venture to speak up— what he managed to say in a few well-chosen words was always pertinent and worthwhile.

I also encouraged Geoff to work with me in the homeless program at my church in Beverly Hills, where I was a volunteer on Monday afternoons. But helping to serve food was too taxing and required coordination he no longer had. I brought him with me on two occasions and he sat on the sidelines while I worked, which only served to remind him of his frustrating experience at the HIV/AIDS food distribution warehouse.

It was aggravating for Geoff that he no longer had a social outlet that didn't involve me. I was always present, always assisting, always trying to make everything we did seem "normal" when it wasn't. Sometimes when we were with friends, I would anticipate what Geoff wanted to say and jump in to say it for him—how I tried not to do that! Or I would guide the conversation in a direction that would give him a chance to respond with a story I knew he wanted to tell—but it was all too artificial. He felt patronized.

At home he showed his resentment. Nothing I did pleased or satisfied him. He bullied and tested me. He was curt, short tempered and sullen, occasionally telling me to shut up and leave him alone. He claimed I did nothing but criticize him. No amount of gentle humor or reassurance dissuaded him. He claimed I no longer loved him, that I wanted him dead. He accused me of lying and working against him. He would sulk in restaurants and other public places when he felt out of his depth or unable to function as he'd like. At night, he had trouble rolling over or adjusting his position in bed, which meant he didn't sleep well and was tired during the day, adding to his irritability.

I knew he was overwhelmed by the rapid decline in his physical condition, but he wouldn't talk with me about it. Too often these abrupt changes came as a surprise to both of us. One day, when he'd been particularly moody, he swiped a bowl of soup onto the floor only seconds after I placed it on the table. I got angry, then realized afterward that he'd only been reaching for the bowl and couldn't control his hand movement. He, of course, was living with frightening changes he couldn't comprehend. He didn't know what would happen to him next.

Knowing he was taking a prescription drug for memory and cognitive loss affected him deeply. Compounding the problem was an odd speech pattern he'd developed. He was no longer slurring his words, but when he became agitated he'd rapidly repeat phrases three times.

"I'm hungry, I'm hungry, I'm hungry."

"No more, no more, no more."

"Don't make me talk, don't make me talk, don't make me talk."

The first time this happened, I was driving to a grocery store. Geoff startled me by shouting, "Take me home, take home, take me home."

I pulled to the side of the road and tried to take his hand to calm him, but he didn't want to be touched. I sat motionless, waiting for his agitation to pass, shaken by the thought that this outburst could have happened in a public place. I couldn't imagine what had prompted the behavior. What if he'd been in this state and tried to open the car door while we were moving—or wanted to get off an airplane? We'd taken another alarming turn, reached another level of inappropriate conduct that I didn't know how to cope with.

One evening while I was washing up after dinner, Geoff banged his hand on the table and said, "You hate me, you hate me, you hate me."

I put my hand on his and said, "I love you, I love you, I love you! Now stop that!"

He angrily pulled away and began shouting at me. I burst into tears. "What makes you do this? Why make me feel bad?" Instead of answering, he stared sullenly at the floor.

I walked him into the den so he could watch television. A few minutes later when I joined him on the couch, he was calm and content to have me sitting next to him. My anxiety increased, imagining myself dealing with this erratic behavior in public. How could I reach him? Settle him down? He seemed unable to control his outbursts and unaware of his actions.

During a flight to New York a few weeks later, a passenger walking up the aisle knocked Geoff's arm, causing him to spill a cup of water. Geoff was enraged that the man didn't stop to apologize. He became agitated, waving his arms and shouting at the man. A passenger seated in the aisle across from us caught Geoff's arm and leaned close, speaking to him in a low, calming voice that soothed Geoff and made him smile. I couldn't hear what the man said, but I was grateful for his intervention.

I mopped up the water, trying to remain calm myself, but I was trembling. I had visions of Geoff trussed and gagged, his hands bound while the pilot made an emergency landing. No allowances are given to unruly passengers aboard an aircraft. An inflight incident that gets out of hand can end in tragedy—and has.

A major turning point occurred in November 2008 during our visit to another neurologist in Los Angeles. Geoff permitted me to accompany him into the examining room. Dr. E put Geoff through a series of tasks, such as drawing circles and hash marks on a page, walking the length of the corridor unassisted and doing various exercises with his hands, feet and eyes.

At one point, while Geoff was performing one of the tasks, Dr. E turned to me and asked if we had "home help." I blinked and said no, that I was able to manage on my own.

He said, "You'll soon need it . . . It might be best to start looking for someone."

As we left his office, Dr. E handed me a flier for the Atypical Parkinsonian Disorders Support Group of Southern California, on which he had circled CBD—*Corticobasal Degeneraton*.

"Is this what Geoff has?" I asked.

"I believe so, yes. Or it could be PSP. I would encourage you to attend the group and find out more about it. Unfortunately there's no treatment at present, but they can offer support and information."

As Geoff and I rode down the elevator, it occurred to me that the doctor had addressed his remarks exclusively to me. Other than speaking to Geoff while he was examining him, the doctor's comments and instructions had been meant for me.

When I got home, I looked up corticobasal degeneration on the Internet and found various descriptions of a rare neurological disease associated with progressive brain degeneration. Initial symptoms included stiffness; shaky, slow or clumsy movements; difficulty with speech and comprehension; difficulty controlling muscles of the face and mouth; difficulty walking and balancing; and short-term memory problems, such as repeating questions or misplacing objects.

I sat stunned, letting the ramifications of Geoff's condition sink in. There was no treatment available. The disease usually progressed slowly over a period of six to eight years. Death was generally caused by pneumonia or other complications. How long did we have? Geoff showed signs of all the symptoms, but when did they start? Stiffness, slurring, balance problems and frequent falls had been noticeable three years earlier, the first real indications that something was wrong. I recalled those odd bits of behavior that had registered years earlier as nothing more than idiosyncrasies: tapping surfaces three times before setting something down, or swatting his hand in front of his eyeglasses as though clearing away debris.

How often had I complained of his tunnel vision, telling him he didn't see something unless "it's right in front of your nose"? Why hadn't I noticed sooner that his peripheral vision was impaired and he was unable to shift his eyes up or down? I didn't want to think back too far, already calculating that he'd had these symptoms perhaps four to five years. Maybe more. It was a timeline I didn't want to consider.

I moved the cursor down the page to the case studies and personal stories, choking up as I read what was in store for someone with these prime-of-life diseases. Then I heard Geoff ease himself into an armchair in the corner of my office. I brushed tears off my face and quickly left the website.

"Are you going to attend this support group?" Geoff asked. I told him I probably would. He laughed and said, "Better you than me. I prefer the bliss of denial."

I smiled. "Well, I was just reading up on it. Really, it's not that bad. We just have to keep you from falling, that's all. Don't worry."

"I'm not. At least you can tell people I don't have Parkinson's or Alzheimer's. They'll never figure out what that other thing is."

No, I thought, unless they have computers. "I won't say anything you don't want me to, that's a promise."

"Good. Besides, there are worse things. It won't be anything we can't handle."

That's as close as the two of us came to talking about CBD. Geoff was aware that he had some sort of neurological condition, and I knew he had to have an even better idea than I did of what was ahead for us. He'd nursed Barbara through her twelve-year bout with MS. Barbara's younger brother had died from ALS. I couldn't blame Geoff for seeking the "bliss of denial," knowing he suffered from another ailment for which there was no cure.

Attending a support group filled me with dread, yet I went. I arrived early. The meeting room in the basement of a hospital on South La Cienega Boulevard was empty but brightly lit. I unfolded a metal chair from a stack propped against the wall and sat down—then immediately stood up again. Shaking with panic, my stomach churning, I headed for the door. I couldn't stay. I'd come back another time. On my way out, I passed a table with reading material on PSP/CBD and took one of the booklets.

By the time I got off the elevator, I was feeling so lightheaded that I sat for a few minutes in a quiet atrium situated off the lobby entrance. After a few deep breaths and some reflection, I knew it wasn't just the meeting I wanted to flee, but the horrible, painful, unthinkable realization of what was ahead for us. I just didn't want to know. I didn't want to face it.

I sat for several minutes watching other people arrive, some using walkers, others being pushed in wheelchairs. A middle-aged couple moved toward the elevator, the woman gripping the man's arm the way I held Geoff's. His face was stony. She was smiling, her face animated. They looked like us, as Geoff and I must appear to other people. I watched them move down the hallway toward the elevator, his gait unsteady, hesitant. I saw the strength in her shoulders, the thrust of her body as she urged him forward.

If she could manage to sit through this meeting, learning the worst and how to cope with it, why couldn't I? I let the elevator doors close and stood for another moment or two before heading back downstairs to the meeting.

The room was now crowded. More chairs were unfolded and scraped into place, then the buzz and chatter silenced as a petite, middle-aged woman stepped to the podium. I panicked again and as I stood up, ready to walk out, the woman at the podium caught my eye and said, "Well, let's start with you. Please, tell us your name and why you've joined us today."

"I'm not really going to stay," I said, and cleared my throat. Then I choked up and the tears came. I could not speak, could not catch my breath.

A young woman took my arm and led me out of the room. I followed her into the hallway, apologizing profusely. "Sorry," I kept saying. "This isn't for me. I shouldn't have come." I knew how demoralizing my behavior was for everyone else in the group and told her that I would leave.

"Everyone feels that way at first. Let's just talk a minute."

The young woman was Welsh and spoke in a lilting accent about her father, who had PSP, progressive supranuclear palsy. I told her I'd never heard about any of these conditions before, that it was hard for me to think of my husband in the advanced stages I'd just seen—then I started crying again. Thank God, Geoff hadn't come with me!

Eventually the young woman and I returned to the room and sat together in the back row. After the meeting, I chatted with the woman who'd been at the podium, a nurse whose husband, a doctor, had recently died from PSP. She was kind and supportive, urging me to come to the next meeting. "It will help you to cope, you know."

I cried in the car all the way home, certain I wouldn't go back for another session. Why couldn't I get a grip on this? If I could keep Geoff safe, take really good care of him, he'd have years—*years*! Maybe there'd be a cure. Maybe he'd go into remission. We'd be normal again.

When I got home, Geoff asked me how it went. "Fine," I said. "Nice people."

"Good. Find out all you can—but don't tell me!" He laughed.

I laughed, too, and told him that I probably wouldn't bother going again.

But I'd witnessed the nature of Geoff's condition in the flesh and saw what we were facing. My attitude had to change. We were not dealing with temporary impairment. This was not fixable. All the time I'd been trying to preserve normalcy, I'd been expecting more of Geoff than he would ever be capable of again. I couldn't waste our time together (five, six years, perhaps!) by pretending this would all go away.

I promised myself not to let his frustration and irritation get to me, or show frustration and irritation in turn. I stopped chiding him about table manners. When he thrashed in bed, I helped him roll over and tucked pillows around him for safety and comfort. I squeezed toothpaste onto his brush and poured water into a cup for him. I cut his food into bite-size pieces, thankful that he could still enjoy food.

Every task we'd once shared became solely my job. I took on certain responsibilities that Geoff had always handled, such as our personal finances. Our accountant had called to ask why a quarterly tax payment had been missed. I thought there'd been a mistake, because Geoff was fastidious about paying everything on time—but then I went into his office and saw the pile of unopened mail on his desk. I'd taken it as a "guy thing" that Geoff had free run of my office but would never let me near his desk—until that afternoon, when I learned that the tax payment had been missed.

I picked up a letter opener and set to work. I found not only the quarterly tax statement, but several insur-

ance premiums due for payment. Why hadn't I fully recognized the implications of Geoff's inability to coordinate his hands? He was as sharp and astute about
finance as ever, but why hadn't I paid attention to the
consequences of his inability to open envelopes or sign
his name legibly?

I began spending an hour or so every morning at
his desk, helping him with his work before going into
my office to do my own. He hated having me "nosing
around"—and his way of doing things was not at all my
way of doing things. I could only recall my recent experience with my mother. He resented having me in his office as much as my mother had resented me in her
kitchen!

"Staff" was no longer just a fun nickname. But as
Geoff relied on me more and more, it also gave me an
opportunity to learn about matters I would someday be
handling entirely on my own.

Geoff's symptoms became so apparent that I began
telling close friends and family about his progressive
neurological condition. He knew that people were calling or taking me aside to ask if he was all right. "Just tell
them I don't have Parkinson's or Alzheimer's," he'd say,
"and be vague."

I avoided using the term corticobasal degeneration,
but anyone could look up CBD or PSP on the Internet
and see the prognosis for a disease that had no cure or
treatment.

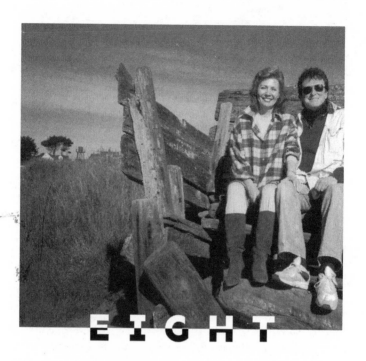

EIGHT

"THERE'S A CABIN
IN THE PINES"

We'd missed a year taking what had become our annual Thanksgiving pilgrimage up the California coast, and Geoff was eager to get back on the road. From its inception, *Los Angeles* magazine had been a reflection of Geoff's love for California. He enjoyed planning our route, mixing favorite stops with new hotels, restaurants and resorts. This time the two of us planned the trip together, choosing a leisurely route since I would be doing all the driving. Surprisingly, it was Geoff's suggestion that we request handicap-equipped rooms whenever possible.

"They didn't exist when I took Barbara on these trips," he said. "I'd like to try them out." If he had still been editing the magazine, there would have been an issue featuring a guide to handicap-equipped travel.

In Cambria, we reserved an ocean-view room that was fitted out with handicap features. Geoff stayed in the car while I unloaded everything. It gave me a start when I saw the "handicap" logo on the door, but when I checked out the "roll-in" shower I felt nothing but relief.

Another night, we stayed at a beautiful rustic inn, but their one handicap-equipped room was already occupied. As comfortable as our standard room was, it would have been foolhardy for Geoff to bathe in its "deluxe spa." The days when we'd light a candle, pour wine and luxuriate together in a Jacuzzi were long over. Instead, I suggested we get an early start and shower before dinner at our next stop, where we'd booked a room with handicap facilities.

The day before Thanksgiving 2008, Geoff and I shared a picnic lunch in Big Sur on a wooded bluff overlooking the Pacific Ocean. There was a chilly drizzle, but we'd dressed for the weather in waterproof jackets with hoods. We had the woods to ourselves and took our time walking along a spongy path of pine needles to find the best spot for our picnic. After finding the perfect view of rocks and surf, we settled on a moss-covered bench under a thick canopy of pine boughs we hoped would keep us dry. I opened wine and set out our spread of salami, cheese, apples, mustard and bis-cuits. We ate in silence for a while, listening to the rush of water nearby and watching a plump seagull edge clos-er, eyeing our picnic basket.

We laughed as the seagull cocked his head, sizing us up. "It's the same fella," Geoff said. "I'd recognize him anywhere."

Geoff was convinced that the same seagull re-turned annually to lunch with us. For more than fifteen years we'd made our annual trip on Highway One up the coast of California to Mendocino, taking a full week for the drive. Eventually we'd reach Big Sur and pull into Grandpa Deetjen's rustic inn, where *I Jesu Navn*, the Norwegian table prayer, hangs on the dining room wall. We'd take a cabin in the woods, complete with a resident cat. The next morning, we'd hike up into the hills, with Geoff carrying a knapsack that I'd stocked with champagne, sausage, bread, cheese and chocolate.

Halfway up the trail, where the path narrows, there's a creek with rushing water. Geoff would wedge a champagne bottle in among the rocks to cool in the icy stream while we walked to the top of the hill. We'd look around, eat some chocolate and then walk back down and sit on boulders to drink champagne, eat our lunch and watch birds swoop high over the Pacific.

Geoff would toss some breadcrumbs and, of course, a seagull arrived—*his* pigeon. He'd throw more bread-crumbs with each new arrival, and more . . . and more— and many breadcrumbs later we would have to flee the swarm of seagulls swooping dangerously around us like a scene out of Hitchcock's *The Birds*.

Unlike our past energetic hikes and elaborate Thanksgiving picnics, our trip in 2008 involved a slow, short walk and food spread on a lichen-encrusted bench—but at least Geoff's seagull had found us.

"We should come in the summer," Geoff said.

I agreed. But in the back of my mind I was already wondering if this might be the last time we'd manage our Thanksgiving drive up the coast.

Days after our return from Northern California, Geoff and I attended a memorial at Chez Jay for its owner, Jay Fiondella, who had died of Parkinson's disease earlier in the year. The ramshackle dining spot on Ocean Avenue across from the Santa Monica Pier had been Geoff's favorite watering hole since Jay opened his eatery in 1960, the same year Geoff launched *Los Angeles* magazine. Its seaside shanty décor featured peanut shells on the floor and red vinyl booths with checkered cloths. We'd celebrated many birthdays and anniversaries at Chez Jay, usually dining on the signature steak au poivre and banana-laced home fries.

On this sad occasion, we presented Mike Anderson, who'd worked with Jay for thirty years and become a partner in Chez Jay, with a framed lithograph by our friend, artist Harry McCormick, featuring Geoff in his safari jacket standing at the bar. Mike was very touched. Afterward, we sat at one of the tables talking with Mike, who asked Geoff to be on his committee to celebrate the fiftieth anniversary of Chez Jay. Geoff was delighted to accept.

We knew many of the other guests at Jay's memorial, too, and stayed until the small restaurant became quite crowded. Then, as we were leaving the party, I tried to help Geoff stand up. We both fell over, toppling tables and chairs, sending wine glasses and peanuts flying everywhere. People rushed to help us back onto our feet, including Mike, who walked us to our car. We laughed and joked, but we were both humiliated and kept apologizing to Mike.

"It was my fault," I said. "My feet weren't planted right."

"Everyone saw," Geoff said. "Just tell them we're drunk."

"I did," Mike said, laughing and clapping his arm around Geoff's shoulders. "But they'd already figured that out!"

We had another event to attend that evening and probably should have stayed home. But it was a holiday party for our homeowners' association and we were board members. We changed out of our wine-stained clothing and went. Both of us were still depressed and shaken from the fall that afternoon. I kept a very self-conscious grip on Geoff's arm. It didn't help matters that one of the other guests, a ninety-two-year-old woman who romped around like someone half her age, told Geoff he ought to get a walking stick instead of hanging on to me.

Neither of us could seem to shake it off. I awoke several times in the night, each time replaying the disastrous tumble at Chez Jay. I'd been so proud and confident of my ability to use leverage to hoist Geoff to his feet. I was convinced I did it so naturally and easily that nobody noticed how much assistance I was giving him. We thought we were terrific, that we fooled everyone, and called it the "Fred and Ginger thing." But for days afterward, we made odd references to "the Chez Jay thing."

"How many people do you think we soaked in red wine?" Geoff asked. "I'll bet we took out at least four tables, easily. How soon do we dare go back for dinner?" I wondered the same thing and wrote Mike a note of apology.

Before leaving on our two-week holiday in New York, we held a "family" Christmas dinner for Geoff's stepchildren and several of our closest friends. I served smoked salmon, short ribs with roasted root vegetables and tarte tatin. The table was set with my mother's china, our best crystal and silver, and a pewter pot overflowing with late-blooming roses and hydrangeas from our garden. We'd shopped for presents for everyone in a neighborhood bookstore, which had become our custom.

I sat with Geoff at the head of the table, wondering if this would be our last Christmas when he could sit comfortably, talk and fully participate in the celebration. Thoughts like these were a reminder to make the most of each moment we had together, but they also made me fearful and anxious. The day-to-day uncertainty was stressful, and so was the dread and panic I felt whenever I thought about what was ahead. Sometimes, when these feelings became overwhelming, I'd sit in the kitchen by myself or walk in the garden and let the tears flow.

But what about Geoff? If I was feeling these emotions, what must his despair be like? Was he experiencing pain or discomfort that I wasn't aware of? Did he dwell on what was ahead? Those thoughts were upsetting to me, yet I couldn't talk to him about my concerns. We were together nearly twenty-four hours a day, but the time was somehow never right to bring up these questions. Nor could we manage to talk about the more practical concerns of his long-term care, or how to organize our finances to handle what was ahead. I suggested we discuss these things with a counselor, but Geoff said it wasn't necessary. "It's not for me, not something I care to do."

Surprisingly, it was the elderly doctor in New York who opened the door to those discussions for us. During our second appointment with Dr. B, Geoff was given a B12 shot and a prescription for yet another medication normally prescribed for Alzheimer's treatment. I took the opportunity to ask the doctor if Geoff really needed this drug, since his memory seemed fine.

"Since I don't have the answers, we're just trying a few things," he explained. "Sometimes drugs serve an off-label purpose, providing a remedy other than the one intended." Because there was no specific treatment for Geoff's condition, the doctor was experimenting with various medications that were available.

"That's fine with me," Geoff said. "I'll be a guinea pig anytime if it means finding something that works." His enthusiastic response probably had much to do with relief at hearing that he wasn't "losing his marbles."

Under the pretext of talking about the precarious lives of musicians on the road during the swing era, the doctor managed to introduce the subject of health directives—"and, while you're at it, setting up a power of attorney. You two should talk over some things so there's no confusion down the road."

To my relief, Geoff agreed. I made an appointment with an estate planner to codify arrangements we already had in place for our separate and comingled finances, and to set up a living trust. The discussions that ensued forced us to face realities and what-ifs that we didn't really want to address, but at the end of the session I sensed Geoff's satisfaction that we'd dealt with these issues. A meeting in an attorney's office had provided us with the forum and structure to express things that needed to be said. I now knew how he wanted me to handle matters, including his last wishes. Then we had a nice lunch with good wine and lots of laughter.

With the new medication and the stimulation of New York, we imagined that Geoff's gait was improving, that his voice was growing stronger. But the reality was no more solo cab rides or walks by himself. I was glued to his side. I had safety bars installed in the bathroom, but showering was still a big undertaking. Well before I turned the faucets on, I prepared carefully, visualizing the whole procedure in my mind and trying to think of everything that could go wrong before it did.

The process took a full hour every morning, and there was not a moment when I wasn't anticipating the next move, careful not to let Geoff slip and fall. Once he was bathed, dressed and seated in the living room watching television, I stepped into the shower myself, shivering with stress.

It snowed heavily, so we stayed in for two days. I read aloud from a book on Sara and Gerald Murphy, part of Geoff's preparation for his Plato Society presentation on the Jazz Age. It was then that he told me about his first trip to the Riviera in his late twenties, when he and photographer Julian Wasser were invited to stay in the home of a French art dealer they'd met in Los Angeles. Geoff, who was passionate about Scott Fitzgerald's writings, set out to track down the villas where Scott and Zelda had lived in the early 1920s. It wasn't until the trip was nearly over that Geoff discovered that the rundown home where they'd been staying was one of the first villas the Fitzgeralds had rented. I urged him to incorporate the story in his presentation.

As I continued to read the biography aloud, Geoff would stop me every once in a while to point out a picture or some piece of Art Deco in our apartment that gave him particular pleasure. There was more to it, of course. I had the impression he was memorizing everything in case he couldn't manage another visit to New York. He was aware that our next trip would be that much more difficult for him.

On the third day, despite the cold, I bundled him up and took him to get a haircut, manicure and pedicure. He loved the pampering. The hairdresser and manicurist were both solicitous, helping me get his coat and gloves on. His left hand was almost useless, so each finger had to be guided into the glove. Then, when I'd think the job was finished, I'd find two fingers jammed together in one space, another hanging limp and empty. Geoff would watch me trying to maneuver his fingers and laugh at my frustration. Mittens were the answer. My sister-in-law Kari sent a fine pair of black suede, lambskin-lined mittens as a Christmas present, along with her homemade peanut brittle. Problem solved.

I missed my mother and our customary family celebration in Minneapolis, but Geoff and I were intent on making the best of Christmas on our own. The new café on the corner of our street, very posh and elegant, had a beautiful *kransekake* on their marble dessert counter. The perfectly decorated almond cake, with looped icing and Norwegian flags, had been homemade by a parishioner from the Norwegian Seamen's Church two blocks away. Mother would have been delighted.

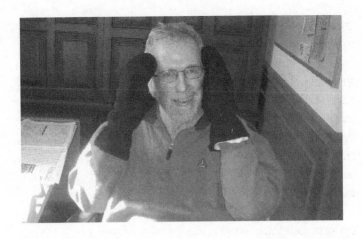

Then, complete serendipity! In the late afternoon I walked to the corner wine shop and saw a leaflet on the counter announcing the annual Christmas caroling at Irving Berlin's house on Beekman Place. Geoff and I had walked past the Berlin house many times, a five-story mansion near the East River. I brought the flier home to Geoff and suggested that we join the carolers, who were meeting in the Katharine Hepburn Room at the Beekman Tower, and stroll with them to the Berlin house. It seemed like a fun neighborhood tradition. Geoff was all for it.

We set out just as darkness fell and slowly walked two blocks in a light mist to the Beekman Tower. Wine was served and songbooks passed around. A new song had been written as a tribute to the recently deceased organizer of the annual event, and several professional cabaret singers took the stage to lead us in learning it. We then set out for the Berlin house, which had been acquired by the Grand Duchy of Luxembourg two years after Irving Berlin died at the age of 101 in

1989. We stood holding umbrellas on the street corner next to a tall Christmas tree decorated with sparkling white lights and sang "White Christmas." Then the consul general opened the door and invited us all inside. My heart danced! How could we be so lucky! Geoff squeezed my hand and we went inside.

The whole house was dressed for a party, with a beautifully decorated Christmas tree in the foyer at the foot of a curving staircase. Geoff was thrilled to be in the room where Irving Berlin had composed *Call Me Madam*, the musical about Perle Mesta, the socialite hostess who became, appropriately enough, U.S. Ambassador to Luxembourg. We sang carols, drank mulled wine with sugar cookies and soaked up the atmosphere of this wonderful house that still had the old-world charm and shabby comfort of a real home.

Afterward, Geoff and I walked back to the Beekman Tower for champagne, a light supper and chocolate desserts in the restaurant on the twenty-sixth floor. We sat at a table looking out on glittering rain-soaked Manhattan, listening to a pianist playing Cole Porter, Gershwin—and Berlin. It was perfect. I savored the evening, wanting to memorize every moment of it.

Evenings like this wouldn't come easily anymore. Had it not been for a creaky, ancient elevator, probably installed for Berlin himself, Geoff wouldn't have been able to join the carolers at the top of the spiral staircase. He could barely walk the few blocks home, but it was so romantic sharing an umbrella for that short magical stroll in misty rain.

On New Year's Eve we joined good friends at the Knickerbocker Club on Fifth Avenue at Sixty-Second Street. I wore a long silk skirt with a black velvet jacket and somehow managed to get Geoff dressed in his tux. Again, what a treat! Wonderful music in beautiful surroundings and a delicious dinner followed by a dazzling show of fireworks, which we watched sitting in window seats overlooking Central Park. At the end of the evening, as we were about to leave, I helped Geoff to his feet, wrapped my arms around him, and we swayed to the Cole Porter music.

Our dancing days were over, but how marvelous to have that romantic moment together in each other's arms.

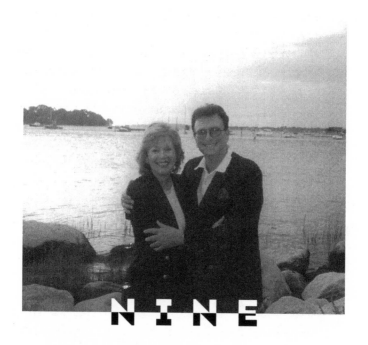

N I N E

"SMILE WHEN THE RAINDROPS FALL"

January 6, 2009—We're off to a good start with our first
Plato Society meeting of the year at UCLA—we'll meet every
Tuesday morning from ten until noon. I'm off to a good start,
too, with a new commercial agent and an audition my second day
back home. I've also managed to set up appointments for Geoff
with the neurologist at Columbia Presbyterian in New York,

and a doctor at the Mayo Clinic. I've already booked our tickets to Minnesota for March 25th.

Dr. B had suggested that I begin keeping a log. "You'll find your notes helpful in tracking the progression and determining how effective these medications are."

I nodded and told him I was already recording information on Geoff's condition in my daily journal. However, I didn't mention that my diary entries were becoming increasingly sporadic and more stilted with the advance of Geoff's disease. I was essentially lying to my own journal! Did I really want to record my whining reactions when Geoff was dealing with far worse setbacks? Owning up to what I was actually feeling was just too hard. I couldn't bring myself to put on paper what sounded like bleak, self-pitying rambles, certainly not when I was at my lowest, just barely coping.

Why admit the reason I'd signed with a new agent was that my former agent dropped me for "booking out" too often? It was a blow I hadn't expected and it hit me hard, particularly as I still had a commercial on the air. My bright and breezy diary entries kept my own brand of denial in place—besides, on the positive side, I was fortunate to have signed with a new, better agent quickly! I also made it clear to my new agents that with travel and doctor appointments, I would have to periodically book out.

Dr. B was insistent that we seek evaluations from both Dr. A at the Mayo Clinic and Dr. F at Columbia Presbyterian to determine conclusively whether Geoff had CBD or PSP. He wrote letters to both doctors on our behalf and provided me with the necessary contact information to make appointments. He also sent me a summary of his findings:

A neurological syndrome characterized by falls, limb kinetic dyspraxia, difficulty with handwriting, increasing difficulty arising from bed or rolling from side to side, along with difficulty dressing. A major feature has been retropulsion resulting in frequent falls. On examination he has difficulty with arising from a chair, manifests moderate ataxia, has evidence of paratonic rigidity of mild degree in all four extremities and has difficulty following alternate limb actions. He has not responded well to Azilect, which was discontinued. He is currently on carbidopa/levodopa. He manifests an extrapyramidal syndrome with Parkinsonian features; however, much of what is present may be evolving progressive supranuclear palsy. I see nothing to suggest a diagnosis of corticobasal syndrome. The impression is that his cognitive function is remarkably intact.

I summarized Dr. B's letter for Geoff: "You hear that? You just have a little case of 'retropulsion' that makes you fall backward."

"Good. Let's hope I've got PSP instead of CBD. I'll take good news where I can get it." He looked very pleased. If he wanted to think having PSP was an improvement on CBD, I wasn't going to discourage him.

We secured an appointment for March 26 with Dr. A at the Mayo Clinic. I booked our flights to Minneapolis and made rental car and hotel reservations for our stay in Rochester. Geoff and I then filled out an exhaustive fifteen-page medical history that told me quite a lot about his heritage. Both paternal grandfathers—one Irish, the other German—had been medical doctors. Family members all seemed to live to a ripe old age except his parents, both smokers, who'd died in their early sixties. Geoff, who had never smoked, had only two chronic ailments: gout and acid reflux, treated respectively with allopurinol and omeprazole.

I was also required to "reconstruct the story" of Geoff's illness, beginning with the first symptoms. I wrote, in part: ... *difficulty getting out of chairs, "plops" when sitting down; ... marked decline in table manners; difficulty cutting food, eating soup; trouble finding things that are in plain sight; doesn't close drawers or cupboard doors; inability to fold or hang clothing or do other common household tasks; ... some inappropriate public behavior, sometimes because of physical inability and occasionally because he's not mindful of being in a public space; ... when agitated, hands shake violently; ... many falls, some serious; difficulty writing, climbing stairs; weeps easily; some cognitive problems, though still sharp with financial planning.*

After jotting down my handwritten statement of symptoms, I decided not to share this section with Geoff. I knew it would seem to him like a "laundry list of complaints" and only upset him—besides, several items sounded like common grievances women generally moaned about, or what I jokingly referred to as "male-pattern sloth." Geoff had seldom pitched in around the house, but now he was unable to help me at all.

I tucked a copy of the Mayo Clinic report into a neatly labeled accordion folder in which I kept insurance information, lists of current and previous medications, all the emergency room reports resulting from Geoff's more serious falls, notarized health directives and power-of-attorney documents, and a handful of CDs with copies of various MRIs and PET scans. I kept the folder on the corner of my desk, ready to grab in case of emergency, a daily reminder of how precarious our lives had become.

I decided to attend another session of the Atypical Parkinsonian Disorders Support Group, primarily to see if anyone else had been to the Mayo Clinic for evaluation. I slipped into a seat in the back of the room, next to a man in a wheelchair who looked familiar to me. After a moment or two I recognized him as Ed Edelman, a highly regarded retired local politician. After the meeting, I struck up a conversation with his wife, who introduced herself as Mari and told me her husband had been diagnosed with CBD. I told them about Geoff and we exchanged cards.

It turned out that some years earlier, Ed, in his capacity as a Los Angeles County supervisor, had presented Geoff with a civic award in connection with *Los Angeles* magazine. I'd seen a photograph of the event framed in Geoff's office. Mari invited us to their home for coffee and I promised to call her to set up a date.

Friday, February 13—We're "fitted" for a stair chair . . . I've known for weeks that we would need to install a chairlift. There's a season for everything, and no denying that for the safety of both of us, I can no longer assist Geoff in climbing the stairs. I showed Geoff the brochure as soon as we returned from New York. His comment: "At least it doesn't look clunky."

I know he was comparing it to the chair lift installed for Barbara some thirty years ago. I said, "Well, someday if we ever need one we'll know where to get it." About a week later, when he stumbled on the stairs and almost fell on me, he said, "I think the sooner the better. How much are they?"

The day before the sales rep arrived to take our order for the stair lift, we happened to drive by a medical supply store. I suggested we stop in to see if there was anything we might find useful. The moment we stepped into the showroom I knew I'd made a mistake. With a glum face, Geoff surveyed the depressing array of walkers, wheelchairs and hospital beds "for sale or rent." I whispered that we didn't need any of this stuff and we left before a sales clerk could approach us.

On the way home, I reminded Geoff that we would be driving to Monterey in a few weeks for Jazz by the Sea. "There's a lot of walking, and those rolling things with the seats might be a good idea when you get tired."

Geoff agreed. "Besides, I wouldn't want to be the only geezer up there without a walker." We both laughed, and I knew the season was upon us. "What color?" I asked. "I'll have the salesman bring along some samples."

Adam, a young, soft-spoken sales rep, arrived with a sample walker called a Classic Cruiser. It was a lightweight model, only eleven pounds, equipped with a wire basket underneath the seat rather than attached to the front handles. I immediately imagined that basket holding our wine and picnic lunch, a book or two and an umbrella when we went on one of our walks. While Geoff tried out the sample walker, Adam and I toured the house and checked out the trouble spots that could be fitted with grip bars and other safety devices. I ordered a lift for the toilet and made note of some of the other items we should install.

When we rejoined Geoff in the living room, he was sitting on the seat of the rolling walker. He'd decided he wanted the Classic Cruiser—in red.

"The cops will see you coming," I warned.

February 14—*Susan, Connell, Bridget and David, old and dear friends, join us for Valentine's dinner—all good cooks! I spend days planning the menu . . . it has to be special. This holiday dinner together has become a tradition. . . . I spend part of the morning and most of the afternoon cooking and setting the*

table, with Geoff sitting at the kitchen table, keeping me compa-
ny. The garden yielded just enough red roses and small calla lil-
ies (in February!) to arrange with greens in a silver bowl.

Our friends arrived with champagne, and the six of
us sat by the fire enjoying hors d'oeuvres. Geoff seemed
completely at ease with our friends, who all knew about
his condition and didn't mention a word about it. I sat
next to Geoff at the dining table, giving him assistance
if he needed it. I'd made his favorite soup, a curried but-
ternut squash with shavings of Granny Smith apple. The
entrée was filet of sea bass on a bed of spinach with baby heirloom tomatoes in white wine, poached in parch-
ment paper pouches tied with strips of thyme from my
garden. Dessert was roasted pear with almond-caramel
ice cream, again one of Geoff's favorites. It was a festive
evening for all of us, made even more special because
Geoff joined in the conversation, laughing and telling
stories. If only this could be our "normal."

We prepared rigorously for Geoff's Plato presentation.
The evening before the big day, we had a run-through
rehearsal. Geoff worried he'd speak too slowly, that
everyone would become impatient. "You've got great an-
ecdotes," I told him, "and nobody tells a story as well as
you do."

I put together handouts for the class and gave Geoff
a master script in large type with highlighted, boldfaced
talking points. Ideally we would have been in separate
discussion groups, but Geoff could not have managed
without my assistance. Given that he needed my help, I
also didn't want to overshadow him. It was tricky know-

ing when to jump to his aid and when to just leave him alone.

In the end, he did a great job. His speech was a bit hesitant, his voice a shade weak, but I only had to give him a few prompts, which I framed in the form of questions. It worked. He was so relieved, and fully deserved the compliments he got from the group after his presentation.

The confidence he gained from that Plato session probably contributed to his willingness to attend the February meeting of the Atypical Parkinsonian Disorders Support Group. Mari called and said she and Ed would attend the Saturday afternoon session if we were going. Geoff wanted to see Ed again—and I'd also mentioned there would be cookies on hand. Geoff would walk on hot coals to reach a cookie jar.

On the drive to the meeting, I filled him in on what to expect. I recalled his comment that he didn't want to meet people in a more advanced state of "deterioration" and "see my future."

I thought about the woman on a respirator who had attended the earlier meeting accompanied by her husband and a nurse. Every few minutes her respirator would emit an unnervingly loud beeping noise. With that in mind, I mentioned to Geoff that there would be people attending the session with types of Parkinson-plus conditions that he did not have, and some would have certain symptoms that he would never experience. I counted on a nice assortment of cookies to see us through.

What I didn't expect, and neither of us was prepared for, was the vast crowd attending the meeting. Word of the Atypical Parkinsonian Disorders Support Group had spread. The room was jammed with close to a hundred people, including patients, family members and caretakers, some of them traveling from out of state. Geoff and I took seats in the back of the room, where Ed and Mari soon joined us.

I gathered up a handful of oatmeal raisin cookies and we attached ourselves to the CBD discussion circle. Ed took over as moderator, and we all introduced ourselves. I quickly calculated that most of the people in our group were men over the age of sixty, and not everyone shared the full range of symptoms. Two men reported memory and cognitive deficiencies before any physical symptoms with speech or movement were apparent.

Ed, whose right hand was contorted and immobile, mentioned that he'd gone to a neurologist when he began having difficulty playing the cello. Geoff brought up his frequent falls, most often falling backward, that led him to see a doctor.

When Geoff also acknowledged his difficulty getting in and out of chairs, an elderly woman seated next to him leaned close and said that her husband, who was eighty-eight years old, "plopped hard" when he sat down, too. Her husband could still climb stairs, she said, but it took great effort. Yet he was "so determined not to be a burden" that he did exercises so he could pull himself up the banister—"but, oh, it takes him a long time." She spoke with pride. "Some of what's wrong is age-related," she said, "but he tries hard despite not having the muscle tone of a younger man."

I tried to guess her age. She was slim and bright-eyed, with close-cropped silver hair, probably in her late seventies, maybe older, but fit and youthful in appearance. Still, she and her husband lived in a two-story house and she was his sole caregiver. As game as she was, I wondered how she could manage on her own when it was hard for me at my age.

"We're doing fine," she said again, as though reading my mind. This time I caught the steely resolve in her voice.

A heavyset man seated next to me said his wife was in a board-and-care facility near their home. "I'm told when you get this condition young, it progresses faster," he said, "and she's only in her fifties. With the dementia and mobility problems, I just couldn't take care of her." He leaned in toward the table, his eyes anxious. "It really came on fast and I don't know what's next . . . how long she might have. Does anyone know?" No one answered, yet the question he raised was undoubtedly on the minds of everyone at the table.

With both patients and caregivers present, there was reluctance to pose certain awkward, more intimate questions. Conversation was polite, restrained and largely anecdotal, with much clearly left unsaid. Geoff would not have tolerated hearing me make any reference to what he called "shortcomings," and it was clear others felt the same way.

With a warning glance to his wife, a man in a wheelchair said, "I don't want to be 'told on,' you know? Nothing's easy."

Another man said he'd stopped driving and "that was hard to give up." Geoff nodded but made no comment.

Ed gently guided the discussion toward positive aspects, such as sharing tips on handicap aids and eligibility for future clinical trials. We didn't linger after the meeting, nor did we talk about the session on our way home. Geoff seemed in good spirits and I wanted to leave well enough alone.

That evening we had dinner with friends, one of them a man who had worked for Geoff at the magazine. We hadn't seen these people in some time and they immediately noticed Geoff's difficulty walking. Geoff told them he had a condition that affected his mobility, then brushed off any further questions. But when we left sometime later, Geoff's legs were stiff from sitting and he stumbled on the doorstep, nearly falling. I steadied him, then helped him into the car with our friends looking on.

"You'll be getting calls tomorrow," he said gloomily, as I pulled away from the curb. He was subdued on the drive home and we barely spoke.

In bed later, I asked, "Everything okay?"

"I just wish this would go away," he said finally. I held him close, wishing all we had to do was just wish it away.

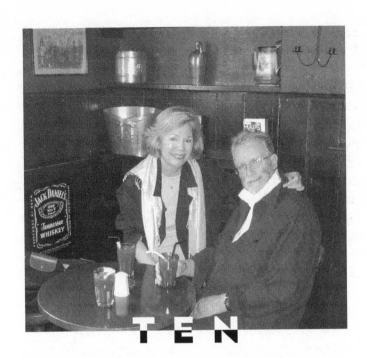

TEN

"MAKE IT ANOTHER OLD FASHIONED, PLEASE"

February 24, 2009—After Plato, I suggest we drive out to the beach for lunch at Chez Jay. The sky is clear blue, the air chilly after a week of hard rain. Mike greets us warmly and shows us Harry McCormick's litho of Geoff that he's hung on the wall. Then Mike sits with us in one of the booths. We order our usual, the famous off-menu BLT. We joke about our *calamitous fall during Jay's memorial, when we toppled three tables, several chairs and many glasses of wine—and laugh loudly when Mike insists, "No one noticed!"*

February 27—Mari and I get together for coffee at Il Fornaio and end up devouring an entire basket of bread, both of us tense, anxious, looking to each other for answers. We stuff our mouths with bread and ask the waiter for more. Ed is older than Geoff and his condition more advanced, but otherwise, Mari and I are dealing with many of the same issues. Ed is on more medications than Geoff, and some lead to constipation and other side effects, all things we would never have brought up in the support group.

She asks if I manage to carve out time for myself—we laugh as we both look at our watches—neither of us can be gone from home more than an hour. We then confide the secret too horrible to tell anyone else—the angry outbursts—ours! I tell her, "Sometimes I just scream, 'Stop, damn it!' when one more thing spills or breaks. It's not his fault, but I can't help myself. I'm always apologizing." Without warning, I burst into tears. Mari says, "I know. I hate it when I shout at Ed, but sometimes I can't take it." There are tears in her eyes, too. I wish I could say that it helps knowing someone else loses her temper. But it doesn't.

Nancy, another one of the women I'd met in the Atypical Parkinsonian Disorders Support Group, called to arrange dinner at an Italian restaurant so we could meet her husband. Josh, a retired entertainment attorney, had a form of Parkinson-plus that had yet to be specifically diagnosed. He had no interest in attending the support meetings but wanted to get together with us. The couple arrived at the restaurant looking very glamorous in a magnificent vintage Aston-Martin roadster, with Josh behind the wheel.

Nancy gave us a jaunty wave as they parked and then hurried around to the driver's side to give Josh a hand getting out of the car. As he and Nancy moved toward us for introductions, it was apparent that even using a cane, Josh had difficulty walking. His left side was stiff, with an arm frozen at an awkward angle, and when he greeted us his speech was noticeably impaired. I could sense Josh sizing Geoff up as we led the way into the restaurant.

"Looks like I'm worse off than you," he said to Geoff when we were seated.

"But you can drive and I had to give it up."

Josh, who had been looking downcast, brightened. "That's one thing I'm not giving up." It turned out he was also not giving up working on his model railroad, an elaborate layout he enthusiastically described as taking up much of their house.

"And the backyard," Nancy added, rolling her eyes. "I'm getting pretty good at helping out."

Josh, a rugged outdoorsman and a tough litigator, said he had not "planned to spend retirement years like this." His frustration evident, he went on to say he hoped for a cure and was open to participating in any clinical trials that were available.

"I wouldn't mind being a guinea pig, either," Geoff said, and I heard the note of determination in his voice.

I listened closely as he and Josh spoke, wondering if Geoff's display of "blissful denial" might have fooled even me. Aside from the occasional outbursts and frustrations with the physical impairment, Geoff appeared accepting of the disease itself. He didn't talk about dying. He wasn't embittered about dashed retirement dreams. His interest in joining a clinical trial seemed to stem more from his need to feel "useful" than a fervent scramble to find a "wonder drug" before it was too late.

I hoped Josh, who was so forthright, would provoke Geoff into revealing inner thoughts he hadn't shared with me. But instead, it was my impression that Geoff smoothed some edges for Josh, commiserating but not lamenting, entertaining the idea of participating in clinical trials, but not to the point of pinning his hopes on a cure.

March 5—*Geoff and I head north for the Monterey Jazz Festival, this time driving a Prius with a red Classic Cruiser stashed in the back seat. Geoff's convertible and my Mercedes sedan are history. On this trip I'm with Geoff all the time, never leaving his side. We still manage to hit all of Geoff's usual haunts, stopping often so Geoff can rest. On Saturday, we leave Monterey for a night in San Francisco. We awaken in our hotel room Sunday morning and I turn on This Week with George Stephanopoulos—shocked to see a friend's photograph pop up in the In Memoriam segment. Jim Bellows! Jim, a fine newspaper editor, and Geoff had known each other for decades, both professionally and socially. He and his wife had come for lunch at our house only weeks ago! Geoff was subdued much of the day.*

March 15—*My brother Orlyn and his wife, Marit, arrive for a brief visit that coincides with the installation of the stair lift. Geoff shows off his new toy ... he loves to climb aboard and ride up, waving like the Queen Mother! We have lunch in Santa Monica and then ride the Ferris Wheel on the pier just for fun. Geoff loves it!*

The stair lift gave Geoff much more freedom and reduced some of my worst anxiety. I'd had frequent nightmares in which I was falling backward down the stairs. In my dreams, my feet, heavy as lead, inched sideways down the stairs, my back braced against the wall,

holding Geoff's arm, each footfall a bit more wobbly . . .
then, a stumble, a slip, a free fall . . . and I would awak-
en, shaking. Or I would dream I was walking behind
Geoff up the stairs, one hand on his back, the other
gripping the banister . . . and suddenly he'd tip backward . . . and I would wake up as we were falling. As
strong and agile as I was, I would not be able to prevent
him from falling or slow the momentum of a fall. I would
end up crushed beneath him.

My nightmares vanished with the installation of the
stair lift but returned after several incidents involving
the car. I'd worked up a reliable routine for helping
Geoff get in and out of the car safely, but occasionally
he'd become impatient and not wait for my assistance.
On one occasion I was still behind the wheel, strapped
into my seat belt, when he opened the door. I managed
to grab his sleeve as he pitched forward. That time, he
only nicked his forehead on the door, but the second
time, he fell out of the car completely. By the time I
could get to him, he was slumped against a parking me-
ter, badly bruised.

One evening, I parked the car on a dark back street
behind a bookstore where our friend, Robert Masello,
had a book signing. I realized I'd parked too far from
the curb and put the car back in gear to pull in closer.
But, in that brief moment, Geoff, who had already un-
hitched his seat belt, released the door handle. The sudden movement of the car caused the door to swing open,
taking Geoff with it. I screamed, turned off the motor
and raced around to find that he'd fallen between the
car and the curb. He'd rolled with the momentum of his
fall so that his shoulder was wedged against a wheel, his
legs splayed under the car.

There was no one around to help us. I struggled on my own to maneuver his legs back onto the curb so I could roll him onto his knees. Using leverage, gripping his hands and pressing my knees against his, I eased him up the side of the car. Eventually I managed to hold him against the car door using my body weight to support him until he regained his footing.

We stood in a tight embrace, my head on his shoulder, until we both stopped shaking. Then Geoff started laughing, making me laugh. We were both filthy but still game for the book signing. I brushed us both down and we managed to arrive before our friend began speaking. After the book signing, we took Robert for dinner. But that night in bed with Geoff lying safely beside me, I couldn't sleep. My mind kept replaying the instant when Geoff fell from the car and the tragedy that could have been.

The night before our flight to Rochester, Minnesota, and our appointment at the Mayo Clinic, I was awake much of the night, anxiously going over the schedule. My brain took a virtual tour of the LAX terminal, imagining the TSA security check and every conceivable mishap we might encounter en route, including snow and ice once we arrived in Minnesota. I realized I'd forgotten to arrange wheelchair assistance at the airports, but hoped we'd be able to manage with the walker. We had snow boots, warm coats. What could go wrong?

We traveled with only one small carry-on roller bag and my handbag, but security was still a nightmare. I managed to get Geoff's shoes and jacket off and sent him through the metal detector while I pushed our coats, the walker, roller bag and my handbag through the screener. When I looked up, Geoff was standing at the metal detector, trying to pull his sweater over his head. I rushed to catch him as he started to topple over, but the TSA staff warned me to stand back.

I was not allowed to assist Geoff in removing the sweater that had a small neck zipper setting off the alarm. Teetering precariously, he yanked off both the sweater and the cotton turtleneck underneath because he couldn't manage to separate the two garments. I watched helplessly as my husband, in his stocking feet, bare to the waist, wearing Dockers without a belt, wobbled through the metal detector. Couldn't they see he needed help?

By the time I made it through the metal detector, Geoff had been force-marched into a holding pen and was tottering on a rubber mat with his arms outstretched. I hurried to give him a hand and was harshly told to move away. Again, I stood by helplessly watching as Geoff, half-naked and shivering with cold, was patted down with a metal wand. Sleep-deprived, anxious and angry, I had all I could do to hold my temper. We weren't even on board yet and I was the one losing it! Finally I was permitted to dress Geoff and gather our belongings.

March 25—*Ahhh, back to the prairie fields of Minnesota . . . cold and snowy, but lovely. I rent a car and we drive to Rochester, arriving in the early afternoon. Geoff and I anticipated a 3-4 day stay at the Mayo Clinic, but finish in one day in under 3 hours! We check out of our hotel in Rochester and drive to Minneapolis, stopping in Bloomington to visit my sister, Sandra. Afterward, we take my brothers and their wives to dinner, then stay the night with Orlyn and Marit. Their gorgeous*

*multi-level house is a treacherous nightmare of stairs and awk-
ward spaces. Geoff is able to brush his teeth, but bathing is out
of the question. After an early lunch with Aunty Pat and my
cousin Glenn the following day, we fly back to Los Angeles.*

The Mayo Clinic is everything one could dream of
in terms of a medical facility—beautifully designed, un-
cluttered, fresh smelling, quiet—and run by an effi-
cient, professional, friendly and caring staff. There was
no waiting. We arrived a few minutes early for the nine
a.m. appointment and were taken directly to an examination suite. Geoff was seen promptly by Dr. A, a tall,
lean, dignified-looking man in a well-tailored suit. During an uninterrupted two-and-a-half-hour session, Geoff
was put through procedures that included an MRI, a
medical exam and neurological testing. He was asked to
blow out an imaginary candle, repeat the letters PTK,
wiggle his tongue, tap his foot and trace letters on his
palm, among many other physical tasks. There was no
sense of being rushed, but no time wasted.

Geoff exhibited symptoms of CBD, according to
Dr. A, who delivered his evaluation in a cool, precise
and detached manner. He told us we would be notified
if there were any clinical trials Geoff might be eligible
to participate in. After we shook hands, Dr. A turned
and walked briskly down the hall and out of our lives.

Geoff and I breezed out of the neurology department as nonchalantly as if we'd been window-shopping
in the Mall of America. We knew pretty much what
we'd already known going in. We were given no new
prescriptions because, as we were once again told, there
was no treatment, no cure for what ailed Geoff.

Meanwhile, all around us in elevators, hallways
and waiting rooms, we saw people in wheelchairs, on

walkers, looking hollow-eyed, pale and wan, wearing hats or scarves to cover hair loss, and exhibiting various other signs of treatments for diseases for which there might be hope of a cure. For Geoff, there would be no surgery, radiation, chemotherapy or life-saving medication. By the time we walked through the lobby, where a pianist was playing show tunes, and stepped out into fresh air, we felt more like we'd accidentally crashed the wrong party than kept a doctor's appointment.

On our drive to Minneapolis, Geoff looked out the window and said, "That wasn't so bad. Nothing we didn't know before—"

"And nothing we can't handle, babe. So, what's next?"

"Travel. Let's just keep moving."

Soon after, we received a thick packet from the Mayo Clinic with Dr. A's final diagnosis: CBD, "unequivocal and diagnostic," with elements of PSP.

Dr. A recommended a bumped-up regimen of carbidopa/levodopa to be taken prior to meals. Otherwise, Geoff continued to take the medications Dr. B had prescribed: mirtazapine (to treat depression) and Exelon patches (to treat dementia, replacing Aricept).

Two weeks after our Mayo Clinic appointment, we cashed in more mileage and headed to New York. I had intended to cancel our appointment with the neurologist at Columbia Presbyterian, but Geoff surprised me by saying he wanted to meet with him. "You never know. Let's see what he comes up with."

I sensed that Geoff, after mulling over the finality of the Mayo Clinic's seemingly quickie evaluation, was feeling let down. For a man as dynamic as he was, it was hard to be told there was no recourse, no hope for a treatment that would slow down the progression. We joked about finding a doctor who would claim, "You know, we've had some success lately with a diet of French fries and butter-pecan ice cream." Another poking and prodding session would be well worth it if we found a doctor who could give Geoff some hope.

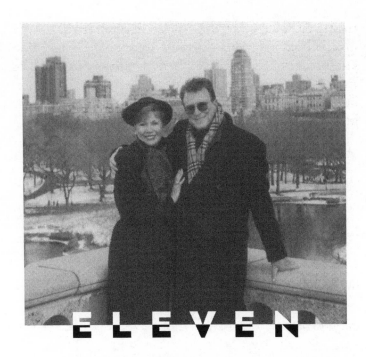

E L E V E N

"I HAPPEN TO LIKE NEW YORK"

It was good to be back in the New York apartment, although it was quickly evident that Geoff's condition had deteriorated in the three months since we'd been there at Christmas. The few handicap aids installed over the holidays were no longer adequate. The toilet was too low, and without wall grips he was stranded without me to help him stand up. He would grab at whatever he could reach, including the towel rack and the edge of the glass shower door.

Once again I realized how fortunate we were to have the means to make all the necessary adjustments in our lifestyle to accommodate Geoff's needs. I bought grip bars and a riser for the toilet. Geoff appreciated the safety features, but at the same time was upset that visitors would see handicap equipment. I assured him that most of our friends were probably installing grip bars, too.

My biggest concern was bathing him. My stomach jumped at the thought of Geoff, soapy and wet, slipping and cracking his head on metal and porcelain as he fell. My brain kept flashing signals: *Stop! Don't!* I followed my instincts. I would no longer take the chance of assisting Geoff into the shower and having him hold the grab bar while I bathed him, as we'd managed to do over the Christmas holidays. Instead I placed a shower mat and a stool on the floor in front of the kitchen sink. I would bathe him, then help him stand up and press my body against his back to keep him stable while I washed his hair using the shower spray on the faucet.

"Sorry," he said, as I was helping him get dressed. "This can't be much fun."

"More fun than taking a chance," I said. "Do you mind not taking showers while we're here?"

"No, it's better." He looked at me and I could see his relief. "Sometimes I get dizzy when I'm standing and have to close my eyes."

Then I realized how frightening it had to have been for him in the shower, trying to keep his eyes open with water streaming down his face. Why hadn't he said something sooner? More than ever, I made a point of planning and mentally rehearsing every movement, every excursion with Geoff so we wouldn't have mishaps.

Dining out had become more important because it provided us with a reason to leave the apartment and give each other undivided attention. I could understand why Geoff loved being with me in the New York apartment; he didn't feel isolated with me working in another room. We could also walk almost anywhere we wanted to go. We dined at neighborhood restaurants where we were known and could get an out-of-the-way corner table. I could cut Geoff's food and help him in and out of a chair without attracting attention.

Before our April 13 appointment with the neurologist at Columbia Presbyterian, we spent an afternoon filling out another lengthy, precise medical history. In answering a series of questions about weight gain/loss, I referred to the folder with Geoff's medical records and made a discovery.

Current weight: 180 *pounds*. Weight three months ago: 190 (*Dr. B's report*). Weight one year ago: 205 *pounds* (*Dr. S's report, April 2008*).

I hadn't paid attention to how much weight Geoff had lost, although we'd noticed he could wear shirts and sweaters he hadn't worn in years. Friends commented that he'd lost weight, but we didn't realize he'd lost as much as twenty-five pounds. He'd also lost an inch in height.

The weight loss was surprising. It seemed to me that Geoff's diet had remained much the same. Perhaps because of his difficulties eating and swallowing we hadn't noticed he was consuming smaller portions at each meal. Also, we ate fewer restaurant meals when we were in Los Angeles, and Geoff would drink a glass of wine instead of having a martini. Oddly enough, I was shedding pounds, too, unaware that my eating habits were changing along with his.

Geoff wanted to take the subway to Columbia Presbyterian. Taxis made him too anxious; even wearing a seat belt and gripping the strap didn't make him feel secure. It was also difficult for him to climb in and out of the narrow back seat with the claustrophobic Plexiglas panel facing him. As counterintuitive as it seemed, he felt much more in control stepping into a subway car. Someone always gave him a seat, and he even liked the jostle of people around him.

He mapped out a route from Lexington Avenue and Fifty-Second Street to Times Square, with a change of trains to 168th Street and Broadway. He knew where there were elevators and ramps and convinced me that, if necessary, he could still climb stairs if I gripped his arm. For Geoff, "life as usual" meant as few concessions as possible—and I couldn't deny him that. Besides saving ourselves a hefty cab fare, we probably made the long journey in less time.

Dr. F, the youngest of the doctors we'd met with, was charming, personable and followed a familiar protocol in examining Geoff. In what seemed nothing more than an amiable chat about travel, music, the stock market and magazine publishing, he got Geoff to recall incidents when he'd fallen or had difficulties sitting, standing, writing or reading. Geoff's responses were good-natured, often humorous, but brief, sometimes hesitant, as though he had memorized the answers and was trying to recall them. He would turn to me, urging me to elaborate. Occasionally I'd give him a prompt, but usually I'd say, "No, you go ahead."

Soon after the session began, I shifted my chair so that I was seated slightly behind him and he couldn't refer to me as easily. His discomfort at not being able to look to me for answers was apparent. I placed my hand on the back of his shoulder for encouragement. Within eighteen months, we'd progressed from Geoff not wanting me in the examining room to his relying on me being with him at all times.

When Geoff performed the various neurological tests, I could see how much he had declined physically since our trip to the Mayo Clinic only a month earlier. Geoff was aware of it, too, and tried to laugh off his complete inability to get out of a chair unassisted. His gait was unsteady and he listed to the right when he walked down the hallway. He could rapidly tap one foot, but not the other. He couldn't write his name legibly, clap his hands or touch his nose with his finger. He accurately drew numerals on a clock face, but a preschooler could have done the same more swiftly and precisely.

While Dr. F covered much the same ground as Dr. A had at the Mayo Clinic, he seemed to dwell more on cognitive tests. I sat off to the side, silently willing Geoff to rattle off the answers that were streaming through my brain. The man who loved language, whose career was spent editing a magazine, couldn't come up with more than two words that started with the letter B. I choked up when he was unable to recall "tree, chair, dog" after Dr. F asked him to recall the three words he'd spoken only minutes before. Geoff, who was addicted to cable news, forgot Bill Clinton when asked to name the last five U.S. presidents.

After a two-and-a-half-hour session, Dr. F concluded that Geoff's condition indicated CBD, but said the progression seemed to be slow moving if, indeed, he'd been showing symptoms for a couple of years. He agreed with Dr. A that we should increase the Sinemet (carbidopa/levodopa) dosage to see if it made a difference, then discontinue if there wasn't a marked improvement.

As we were leaving his office, Dr. F told Geoff, "The main thing you need to do is stay safe and not fall. Within the time frame for CBD, you're doing well. If you've had falls and other symptoms for five, six years, I would have expected to see greater deterioration by now."

Geoff was quick to pick up on the reference to a time frame for CBD. "I think Kathryn has kept that from me," Geoff said. "If there's a time frame for this thing, how long are we talking about?"

So much for denial! I was surprised he'd asked—or wanted to know. Before Dr. F could respond, I jumped in and said, "Who knows? Everyone's different. The fact that you're in otherwise good health is probably slowing the progression. If you had diabetes or emphysema, everything would be more complicated."

Dr. F backed me up. "You're doing better than most. Just don't take a bad fall, because that could change everything."

"I just wondered," Geoff said. "I feel good, but I seem to be going downhill pretty fast."

Geoff knew I'd curtailed any direct answer about life expectancy with CBD. But I didn't want to hear the "six to eight years from diagnosis" answer, either. Why rob ourselves of the present by worrying about a ticking clock and a future over which we had no control? I could play the denial card, too.

"What about a drug trial?" I asked. "Is there any kind of treatment program being tested?"

Dr. F suggested putting us in touch with a colleague, Dr. Yvette Bordelon at UCLA. "There's not a great deal of clinical study available on these disorders. But if you're interested in participating in a clinical trial, she might have something going in Los Angeles."

"Great," Geoff said. "I may as well be a guinea pig."

Despite a long, grueling session, we left the consultation in good spirits, which seemed to be our pattern. We knew as much as we could know. There was nothing we could do, other than sign up for a clinical trial and hope Geoff would be accepted. In the meantime, we had life to live. We stepped out of Columbia Presbyterian into misty drizzle and a clog of rush hour congestion. Even traffic and bad weather didn't diminish Geoff's spirits.

"God, I love New York!" he said.

"Are you up for dinner at the National Arts Club?"

"You bet. I'll even go in a cab. And I want a martini."

We huddled under my umbrella for only a minute or two before a taxi pulled up and whisked us down to the club on Gramercy Park. Brian Kellow, an editor at *Opera News*, joined us for dinner and we stayed for a book-signing event afterward. The club was jammed, but we somehow managed to secure three decent seats for a hilarious discussion between Christopher Plummer and Zoe Caldwell tied to Plummer's newly published autobiography. We were thrilled to hear stage veterans Plummer and Caldwell trade theatrical war stories in their plummy accents ("Christopher, darling, please do tell us about your loooong years as a druuuunk!" Caldwell trilled), which turned out to be the perfect antidote to our own looooong afternoon at Columbia Presbyterian.

Within a week, we received a summary from Dr. F, and once again the diagnosis was much as we expected. Dr. F took note of my comments that for at least ten years Geoff would "plop" when sitting and lean to the right when walking. I always walked on Geoff's left side so he wouldn't bump into me. I had also mentioned that Geoff had a history of weeping with little provocation, and that his hands shook when he became agitated. Dr. F wrote:

Most striking was the presence of apraxia, especially involving the left hand. He could hardly perform any specific maneuver, such as finger tapping, hand opening, or pantomime simple tasks, such as hammering or saluting using his left hand . . . there was a hesitancy to his execution of tasks with the right hand, even though he could complete them. . . . Visual fields were full. His gaze upward was minimally decreased, but there was no supranuclear palsy. . . . His speech was slow . . . and had a husky tone. He could not perform rapid movements with the left hand due to apraxia (inability to execute purposeful movements, despite having the desire and the physical ability to perform the movements). . . . He rose from a chair only by propelling himself . . . his walk was brisk, without freezing, made quick turns. Overall, he had some mild abnormalities of ocular motility, dyspraxia, midline cerebellar findings, paratonia, and a range of cognitive deficits including verbal fluency, motor planning and memory. Mr. Miller has been alternatively diagnosed clinically as having corticobasal ganglionic degeneration (CBGD), atypical Parkinsonism, multiple systems atrophy (MSA), and perhaps others. The PET scan was not helpful in making a differentiation. On clinical grounds, the striking dyspraxia does suggest CBGD. . . . It is possible that his Parkin-

sonism syndrome will yet evolve into CBGD or PSP, but the course is much slower than noted. I reviewed the difficulties in making a specific clinical diagnosis. I suggested that he consult with our colleague, Dr. Yvette Bordelon at UCLA, an expert on Parkinsonism, for further consultation. It was a pleasure to meet this charming man and his devoted wife.

"So, what does he say?" Geoff asked.

"He doesn't know exactly what you have, but whatever it is, it's slow moving. He also thinks you're charming, I'm devoted and that we should see another doctor."

Geoff took the news well. His buoyant spirits had much to do with being in New York. In the evenings we'd meet friends for dinner or stop in at Birdland, Sofia or one of the other music venues. When we were in public places, I made a point of looking cheerful and making everything look effortless, because people would then respond with a smile or a friendly gesture, which, in turn, gave Geoff a boost. Appearances mattered because we were treated better when we needed a little extra time maneuvering in restaurants or wanted some help getting through a doorway.

I made even more of an effort with friends because no one would want to be around us if there was any sense of strain or unpleasantness. Some of our friends were going through their own tough times and didn't want to talk about health problems any more than we did. When anyone asked about Geoff, I'd say, "He's doing fine," and leave it at that. Still, no matter how upbeat we were, there were friends who drifted away. Understandably, a few former colleagues of Geoff's found it awkward and difficult to deal with his diminished capacity when they'd known him as such a vital, forceful person.

Before I packed for London, I scoured Macy's men's department for sweatpants with a fly front to make it easier for Geoff to use the cramped toilets on our flight. I found some Nike pants in good quality black cotton with an elastic waist, fly front and zippered pockets that were so well cut it was hard to tell they were sweatpants—and bought two pair on sale.

But no matter how carefully I prepared for the trip, I was awake the entire night before our flight, planning my moves going through security: *Seat Geoff on walker, remove shoes, jacket, place in bins, send Geoff through the metal detector with boarding pass in hand, then fold walker, place on conveyor belt with laptop, handbag and small roller bag, race through, retrieve Geoff, clothe him, check nothing has been left behind and head for the gate.*

The following morning, all went well until the metal tab on the fly front of the swell new Nike pants (I'd been so smug about not having to remove a belt, why didn't I think of that!) set off alarms. By the time I'd made it through the metal detector, Geoff was wobbling in his stocking feet on a rubber mat with his arms stretched out while a security guard ran a wand over his body. Common sense might have indicated that an elderly man using a walker might not be capable of standing on his own. I was warned to keep my distance and had to wait helplessly as Geoff tottered and fell against the guard. Fortunately Geoff was *not* charged with assault or interfering with a security officer! With no further mishaps we boarded our 8:30 a.m. flight to London.

Aboard the aircraft, I remained alert to every conceivable mishap: Geoff falling in the aisle, getting stuck in the toilet, or losing both his dignity and temper and lashing out. On a long flight, anything could happen to cause an incident. If he became frustrated or agitated, he wouldn't be able to control his voice or his hands. I worried that I wouldn't be able to settle him down if his voice got loud, or his speech abusive and repetitive.

He always insisted upon going into the bathroom alone, while I stood outside waiting for him. How would I deal with it if he came out of the cabin with his pants down, angry because he couldn't work the fly? Handling these situations at home or in public places was difficult enough, but how would I deal with it during a seven-hour flight in close quarters with no way out?

Before the aircraft left the terminal, Geoff showed signs of impatience. I buckled his seat belt, gave him a kiss and held his hand. "Just let me know if you need help. I'm here. Want some nuts? Chocolate?"

Throughout the long flight, I spoke gently, took his hand and smiled whenever I sensed Geoff becoming disgruntled or uncomfortable. Fortunately there were no babies crying or children kicking the back of his seat. When Geoff had to go to the bathroom, I didn't take any chances. I forced my way into the cubicle with him. I braced my foot on the washstand, with my knee supporting his back so he couldn't fall backward. Wedged securely, I was able to assist him. The really tricky part was getting the door open again. Thank God for ballet training!

The flight was smooth, the aircraft not crowded. After landing at Heathrow, we made it through passport control and customs without incident—a miracle! The best part was that Ben, my former husband, was waiting for us at the Cottage with chilled wine, music playing and our bed turned down. How does one manage without two husbands?

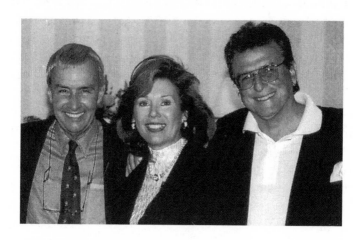

The purpose of the trip to London was to prepare the Cottage for short-term rental through a neighboring boutique hotel. After thirty-nine years, it was time to deal with the overflowing closets and attic. Ben and I spent ten days emptying the two-bedroom house of personal belongings, unearthing forgotten treasures in the attic, and disposing of mementos and furnishings we'd cherished for decades. The décor reflected an early '70s-era time warp, when Victorian glass-globed lamps and Portobello Road bric-a-brac was the fashion. We even had an Aspidistra plant flourishing in a quaint ceramic pot on a bamboo side table—ours was not an IKEA home.

While Geoff watched CNN, Ben and I carted vintage suits, coats, designer dresses and Carnaby Street hippie gear to a nearby antiques dealer, who was thrilled to buy it all. We showed the dealer photographs of the antique furniture in the Cottage and were told, "No one wants brown furniture anymore, mate." But we persevered and found a man with a van and an appetite for old LPs, steamer trunks, oak picture frames, hand-embroidered linens, cookware, a brass bedstead and, indeed, "brown furniture." It was wrenching, but also a relief not to have to manage a house some 5,000 miles away. Whatever we didn't put aside to ship to our respective homes stateside—or couldn't sell, donate or give to friends—found its way to one of Westminster City Council's Big Black Bins. I tried not to look.

Most evenings, we cleaned ourselves up and dined at a neighborhood Italian restaurant. Ben and Geoff had a good deal in common—aside from me! Contentious moments between sparring former spouses dealing with a museum of mistakes, blunders and old wounds were mitigated by Geoff's calming presence and ready humor. There were a few tears, too, thinking back on bygone times and friends no longer with us.

Going through the kitchen cabinets, I came across items I recognized as wedding presents and souvenirs from memorable trips. I also recalled that the cabinets themselves had arrived as unassembled raw wood that we had sanded, stained and installed ourselves. I remembered that when we moved in, a vintage 1920s-era gas cooker was such a mystery to me, I had no idea how it worked. How many times had I repainted the walls, repairing cracks left by German buzz bombs during the war? Inevitably, nostalgia turned to penetrating sadness when I reflected on our present situation. Such a lot was coming to an end.

It was my idea to spend a weekend in Paris, where Geoff and I had celebrated our honeymoon. It was a rash, spur-of-the moment, crazy notion, made slightly less insane because another couple we adore decided to travel with us. We booked seats on the Eurostar and managed to reserve our favorite room in the Lenox, a Left Bank hotel with a great Art Deco jazz-inspired bar enshrined to Louis Armstrong. Without Jo-an and Adrian lending a hand, we couldn't have managed such a trip, but neither did we impose ourselves on them as we packed in museums and fine dining. If this trip marked the end of European travel together and our tenure in the Cottage, we did it in style!

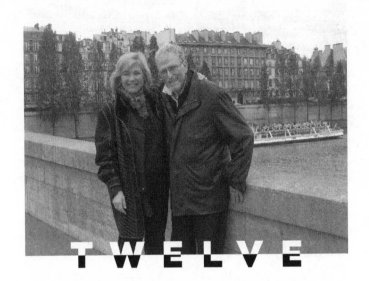

TWELVE

"I REMEMBER IT WELL"

June 5, 2009—*Home again. Roses are blooming. The sun is hot, the pool inviting. Geoff stands on the balcony outside the bedroom door, hanging on to the railing, watching me swim.*

"How is it?" he asks.

"Great!"

I swim back the length of the pool, my eyes suddenly flood-

*ing with tears. I haven't cried in days, but now I can't stop and I
don't want Geoff to see. I dip my head in the water and keep
swimming.*

Geoff loved the pool and swam every day, April
through October. When he was still editing *Los Angeles*
magazine, he'd shake off the tensions of the day by swimming laps when he got home. Weekend afternoons, he'd
swim and then lie by the pool, listening to jazz and
catching up on his reading. In the evenings, we usually
cooked on the outdoor grill and ate our dinner in the
upper garden, looking across the pool, lit up and landscaped with pots of flowering plants along the perimeter. Neither of us wanted to give up dining in the garden
in front of the outdoor fireplace, listening to jazz and
watching the moon rise above the ridges of the canyon.

However, it was becoming more difficult. I tried
to accommodate Geoff's needs by installing handrails
and safety grips, but it still wasn't safe for me to get him
in and out of the pool on my own. I considered installing
ramps and a lift to the upper garden, something Ed and
Mari had done in their garden, but in the meantime we
were able to enjoy the lower patio and pool area. That
afternoon, I surprised Geoff with an early birthday gift,
a sturdy new canvas chair equipped with a side tray for
a snack, a pocket for reading material and a cup holder.

For dinner, I'd planned to grill swordfish to serve
with homemade mango and arugula salsa, another of
Geoff's favorite meals. I helped him into the new chair
and brought him a white wine spritzer in a plastic goblet. I turned on the CD player in the pool house so he
could listen to jazz while I brought the tray with our
dinner out to the grill.

Minutes later, just as I was about to walk back out

of the kitchen, I heard Geoff calling me, his voice sounding odd and distant. Alarmed, I put down the tray and hurried outside. He wasn't sitting in his chair—and I couldn't see him anywhere.

In full-blown panic I shouted his name and raced to the pool to see if he'd fallen in. Then I ran across the little bridge to our bedroom, thinking he might have tried to walk to the bathroom on his own. I heard his voice again, turned back to the garden and spotted him. He was lying partially concealed by shrubbery at the bottom of the steps to the pool house. Stifling a scream, I raced down the walkway and knelt beside him. His body was crumpled sideways, a stream of blood flowing from beneath his head.

"Just get me up," he muttered, his voice cracking. "I'm fine, just get me up."

I gently rolled him toward me, bracing his shoulder against my knee. The plastic goblet I'd used for the spritzer was cracked but still clutched in his hand, the liquid pooling on the walkway. His eyeglasses, bent and broken, were near the steps.

"How did you get way over here?"

"I wanted to turn on the pool lights."

"You should've waited. I wasn't gone five minutes!"

"I didn't want to bother you."

Damn, those words! I wanted to scream, "Please, please bother me!"

Instead, I calmly told him to hold still while I assessed his injuries. I eased his face from the paving stones, feeling for any pulpy flesh. I carefully slid my hand under him, lifting him up gently in case he'd injured his back or broken an arm or ribs. A deep gash oozed blood above his right eye, with cuts and scrapes on the side of his face, nose and cheek. He was bleeding profusely and I was afraid he'd struck his head on the steps while falling.

"I'm calling the paramedics, Geoff. I don't dare raise you up any more."

"Don't call! I'm fine. Get me up."

"Don't move! I'll be right back."

I ran up the steps to the pool house to call 911. I gave the dispatcher my name, address and specifics about Geoff's injuries. "He's breathing. He had a bad fall. He's seventy-one, with a neurological condition. There's a lot of blood. I don't know how badly he's hurt." I didn't say CBD, because I was sure the dispatcher wouldn't know what it was. I should have said Parkinson's to give a clearer idea of his condition, but I didn't.

These thoughts and myriad others raced through my head as I hurried back to Geoff, then raced to unlock the side gate. I punched up Harry's phone number as I ran. Harry answered his cell phone almost immediately. As I ran through the kitchen, grabbing towels on my way back up to Geoff, I told Harry what had happened. "I've called the paramedics. I don't know how bad it is."

"I'm on my way, maybe five minutes."

When I reached Geoff, he was trying to sit up. I raised him only slightly on his side, cradling his head and pressing towels against the flow of blood. He said he felt lightheaded, dizzy. I kept asking him questions, making him answer, afraid he'd lose consciousness. When I heard the siren and the sound of a truck pulling up outside, I shouted, "Side door! Back garden!"

Harry had arrived at the same time as the paramedics and led them down the walkway. I stood back as they examined Geoff, horrified to see how badly his face was injured. I answered questions, telling them what I thought had happened. I explained Geoff's neurological condition and said that he must have got up from his chair the moment I stepped into the kitchen. The plastic glass was still in his hand because he'd been unable to release his grip on it. Carrying it in his good hand, he'd tried to grasp the railing with his stiff hand and had fallen backward down the steps.

While the paramedics tended to Geoff, I hurried to my office to grab the folder containing insurance information, medical records and list of medications. Meanwhile, Harry began closing up the house, checking the kitchen and locking doors. The paramedics secured Geoff in the ambulance and told us he would be taken to the emergency department at UCLA Medical Center. I climbed into my car and followed Harry to the hospital. As I was driving down the canyon, Kay, another close friend, happened to call. When I told her what had happened, she said she would meet me at the hospital later.

By the time Harry and I arrived, Geoff was already in an examining room. His face and arms were swathed in gauze, his body hooked up to monitors. He looked frail and frightened, yet he smiled when he saw me. "Mad at me?" he whispered.

"No, of course not." But I gave him a fierce look and added, "Next time I say 'sit,' don't move, damn it! This didn't need to happen."

"The pool lights. You didn't turn them on. And I wanted to change CDs."

I nodded and smiled, my mouth clamped shut. What could I say? Both had once been effortless tasks for him, but he was no longer capable of changing CDs and would not have been able to reach the switch for the pool lights. Why hadn't he waited for me, *damn it*? I was angry, barely able to contain my rage. We could have been home eating swordfish and watching the *damn* moon rising in the night sky! I knew he couldn't control his impulses or weigh consequences, but that didn't mitigate my fury and frustration. Why hadn't I brought the food out and then seated him in his new chair—*why, why, why*? Short of chaining him down, what was I supposed to do?

I was so *damn* proud of the *damn* chair I'd found that I thought was so *damn* safe and would give him so much pleasure, but I should have known that, left alone, he wouldn't be able to resist the temptation to get up and "set the scene." I imagined every hideous scenario that could have happened. What if he'd fallen in the pool? Broken his back or his neck? Lost an eye falling into the bushes? *Damn!*

Yet all the while I was blaming myself for not being more vigilant, I calmly held his hand and stroked his arm. Did he have any idea what was going through my mind? At the very least, we faced hours in the emergency room, a possible hospital stay and considerable pain and discomfort for Geoff. I was also aware that my anger stemmed from my concern that this mishap was a life changer for both of us. Ringing in my ears was the warning given to me by every doctor, including Dr. F: *Just don't let him fall; it could change everything.* I'd let him fall.

Harry left soon after Kay arrived about an hour later. She stood with me for more than two hours while doctors, nurses and technicians came in and out of the cubicle, a space too narrow to accommodate chairs for us. Kay left around eleven o'clock, but I remained, leaning against a wall, feeling drained, frustrated and completely useless.

Throughout the night, I answered questions, mostly the same questions, while waiting for tests and X-rays to be done, consciously making myself as responsive and accommodating as I could. My mantra—*be nice, smile!*—had everything to do with garnering as much prompt attention and assistance from the emergency room staff as possible.

Around midnight, I wedged a hard plastic chair next to Geoff's gurney and sat with my hand on his arm. While he dozed, I huddled in my corner, listening to the bleeps on the monitors, wondering why not a single hair-raising, stupefying calamity of the sort that occurs five times an hour on ER and *Grey's Anatomy* happened on my watch. I spent close to thirteen hours in a boring, uneventful emergency room, devoid of any distracting drama, craving food and a glass of wine, wishing I'd thought to bring a book and trying very hard to deal with my anger and resentment. *If only I'd chained Geoff to the chair!*

We were released shortly after six a.m. I loaded Geoff into the car and drove home. The June gloom, with its heavy, brooding skies, matched my mood. Geoff, his swollen face bruised and bandaged, smiled and appeared almost ebullient. Odd as this seemed, I'd witnessed this post-trauma euphoria before with Geoff. Perhaps it was relief that the ordeal was behind him and nothing worse had happened.

"How do you feel?"

"Pretty good, no pain. Just hungry." As I turned into Benedict Canyon, Geoff said, "I'm sorry."

"I know. I'm sorry, too. But at least no broken bones. You'll be fine."

"I couldn't help it, you know."

"I know that, too." I rubbed away the salty tears biting my sore, itchy eyes. "I'm sorry, Geoff. I know you know that I was mad. I'm so sorry. You were hurt and had to be more scared than I was. I'm sorry. I love you. I know you understand."

"Couldn't help it," he repeated, a smile still on his lips. "Couldn't help it. Couldn't help it."

I also knew he couldn't help repeating himself. Nor could he resist the impulse that made him get out of the chair. Impaired judgment was part of the syndrome. He couldn't help it that he was unable to put down a cup or glass. He couldn't help not being able to grasp the railing with his bad hand. He couldn't help falling backward. But could I help it that I'd left him alone for five minutes? Yes!

I gave in to emotion on the ride home, any residual anger washing away in a flood of tears I couldn't help. I kept repeating, "I'm so sorry, so sorry!" Meanwhile, in the passenger seat next to me, Geoff sat immobile, his face stoic but for a small smile. The palms of his hands were anchored on his knees in a pose as stony as President Lincoln's in the Lincoln Memorial. Had anything I said registered with him? I could only hope he understood how sorry I was—for *everything*. His unwavering smile and vacant look were enough to make me doubt he even heard me.

I parked in the driveway and hurried to unlock the back door, not wanting to leave Geoff alone a moment longer than necessary. I managed to extricate him from the car and maneuver him into the downstairs guest room, one plodding step after another. By the time I took him to the bathroom, fed him breakfast, removed his clothing, bathed him, gave him some juice and more pain medication, the heavy skies were beginning to brighten. Geoff fell asleep instantly, the hint of a smile still on his lips. It occurred to me that perhaps he couldn't control his smile anymore, either.

In the kitchen I drank a cup of strong tea and confronted the tray with our dinner, a crusted and congealed relic of the night before. I tipped everything into the garbage disposal, poured myself a glass of white wine and took a walk in the upper garden. I passed by the patches of dried blood staining the walkway and picked up Geoff's broken eyeglasses, left behind on a ledge.

I gave in to hot, scalding tears as I tucked them in my pocket. Our lives had changed overnight, and I knew it. I took my time feeling sorry for myself, for Geoff and the heartaches I knew were down the road.

I managed to finish my wine before the gardeners arrived to see me drinking my breakfast. Nor did I want to be around when they hosed down the walkway, wondering at the rivers of brown stains rimming the pool and the footprints imprinted like henna tattoos on the steps. After cleaning up the kitchen, I called to leave a message on the UCLA switchboard that we wouldn't be attending the Plato Society meeting at ten a.m. I hung up the phone wondering if we'd ever again be attending another Plato session. Just how much had our lives changed? Then, feeling the effects of the wine and lack of sleep, I climbed into bed and curled up next to Geoff.

The following day, Geoff's shoulder was causing him considerable pain and discomfort. We made an appointment with an orthopedic surgeon, who diagnosed a fractured shoulder and scheduled surgery. That week, our days were taken up with doctors, home care therapists and long stretches icing Geoff's shoulder. In the evenings we watched movies together, then I read to him until he fell asleep for the night.

June 16—*I can't help but think of my mother on her birthday. I'm also reminded that only two years ago, she celebrated her 93rd birthday, knowing she would never see another year through. If she had, she'd still be driving a car—I've framed her driver's license. Geoff was still driving, too, back then, and could manage to do everything on his own, although there were signs at the time that I didn't fully recognize. What a huge change just in the past nine months. Now, since his fall, Geoff cannot get out of a chair or walk without my help. He can't bathe, brush his teeth or use the toilet on his own. He can't write, read a newspaper or feed himself. He needs me—so stop being impatient! What's so important you can't just sit, hands in lap, and do nothing but give him attention? Stop! Please, no regrets! Remember how it was with Mother. Don't lose him and have to recall the times you were unkind, impatient—or just too busy.*

That entry wasn't the first or only time I admonished myself to be patient and not stockpile regrets. I physically tried to slow myself down—not easy, because I'm a quick person. My fingers fly when I'm cooking, sewing, gardening. I walk fast, eat fast, read fast. Sometimes those quick reflexes worked in my favor caring for Geoff, but I was constantly reminding myself to just sit with him rather than jumping around doing too many things at once. I did not need to entertain him. I just needed to *be there*.

The shoulder surgery was scheduled for June 17 at

2:30 p.m. We arrived at Cedars-Sinai hospital at noon. Geoff, who had been fasting since midnight, was hungry and irritable. Despite having filled out preregistration forms, I was required to fill out the same forms again. Geoff became increasingly impatient waiting in the reception area. I accompanied him into pre-op and, because I knew it would calm him, requested to stay and undress him myself. While he was being "tubed up," I answered questions from one nurse and attendant after another, glad that I had brought the medical folder with abundant photocopies of his medication list and insurance information.

Yet, despite all the checking and double checking I'd done all week, it was discovered only minutes before Geoff was to be wheeled in for surgery that certain X-rays and signed medical forms from Geoff's GP were missing. I cursed Dr. S, the avuncular internist Geoff adored, who had assured me that everything the hospital had requested had been submitted.

The surgeon, anesthesiologist and surgical nurses cooled their heels while the pre-op nurse chatted with the doctor's office staff on speakerphone. Geoff, listening to the exchange broadcast into his pre-op bay and hearing that surgery would have to be postponed several hours, became frightened and agitated. I tried to calm him, finally resorting to the gallows humor he appreciated. I told him the surgeon had left in a huff, but they'd found a replacement, someone who was not actually a doctor but had stayed in a Holiday Inn Express the night before and would be performing surgery with the penknife and tweezers he had in his pocket. I told him it would hurt a whole lot. Geoff laughed and squeezed my hand.

It was 10:30 p.m. before Geoff was finally wheeled out of recovery and into a hospital room for the night. He was subdued and disoriented, his face waxen in the harsh light. His anxious eyes told me I couldn't leave him alone for the night, although that had been the plan. I requested a cot and stayed, holding his hand and listening to him breathe. At six a.m., pale light seeped through the window. Geoff awakened, his smile bright when he saw me.

Geoff's shoulder healed well and he impressed me with his determination to regain strength and mobility. I took him for hour-long physical therapy sessions three times a week and assisted him with daily exercises at home. His incentive was the impending arrival of our good friends from London for their annual summer visit. Geoff was sure that James, young and fit, would be able to get him into the pool, and talked about it incessantly.

The day after James, Trish and their son, Max, arrived, they surprised Geoff with an early birthday gift—a life jacket. I helped Geoff into his bathing trunks and sporty new life jacket, and then James and I maneuvered him down the few steps into the pool. Geoff was ecstatic. The jacket made him so buoyant that with a little assistance he could safely paddle around, which helped him regain even more strength in his limbs. In addition to the daily swim, our friends provided what amounted to two weeks of summer camp, enabling us to go places and do things we couldn't have managed on our own. Also, with all the exercise and wonderful companionship, Geoff was in far better spirits and physical shape by the time they returned to England.

The void left by their departure was immense.

Geoff pined for their return, especially missing young Max, who had shown him such affection. He missed having James help him into the pool and his irreverent "guy talk" and good humor. I tried to buoy Geoff up, but I was feeling down as well. Summer camp was over.

More than that, we'd undergone a huge change because of Geoff's fall. I could feel our world closing in. I almost preferred sleepless nights to the nightmares in which I replayed Geoff's terrible fall and its aftermath.

August 4—*The LOOP that wakes me at night and won't let me sleep always begins with me telling Geoff to stay in the chair. "Don't move. I'll be right back with dinner." But he gets up. He falls. Why didn't he listen to me? Frame by frame, each moment passes through a projector, giving me long minutes to relive every hoary detail. The empty chair. The clutch of terror. Calling his name. Where is he? Drowned? Blood oozing on the cement. Fear. He's not moving. Broken back? Cracked skull? Paramedics. Can't give in to panic. Trembling, hand over insurance cards photocopied on a single page. Why do I feel so proud I can present a list of his medications? Geoff, battered and bloodied, loaded onto a gurney and transported to the ambulance. Anger. This didn't have to happen! Loathing my anger. The hospital vigil; angry again! Geoff smiling; charming the attendants, which I also resent. Vending machine dinner. Craving wine, sleep. Geoff chatty to the attendant pushing his wheelchair—like this has been a social call??? My mind racing—how to get Geoff into the car, the house, the bed. Seeing the remains of our dinner. More anger. This didn't have to happen! Why did I let it happen?*

There was no question that Geoff's fall had shaken both of us. I was certain he was replaying his own loop of the event. He was no longer insistent about doing things on his own. He sat with his hands gripping the cushions or arm rests, as though afraid he might fall out of the chair. As much as his cocky assertiveness had irritated me, I grieved its passing.

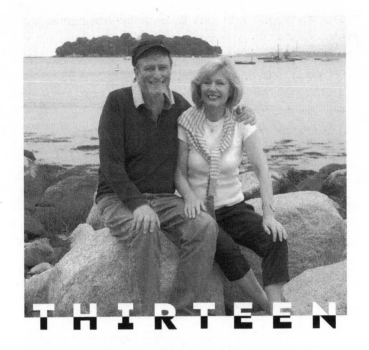

THIRTEEN

"BEGIN THE BEGUIN"

The antidote, as always, was travel. Geoff and I were both heartened by the prospect of spending a month in New York, even in the heat of August. I used the transport chair to wheel him from our apartment to physical therapy sessions at the Columbia Presbyterian facility on Sixtieth Street off Madison Avenue. Afterward, we would stop for lunch somewhere and window shop on our walk home.

We also packed in dinners with friends, evenings at Birdland and the National Arts Club and screenings of films at the Motion Picture Academy's theatre in our neighborhood. One of the highlights of our stay was a trip to the newly renovated Minetta Tavern with our friends from Connecticut, Joel and Hannah Baldwin. I had wonderful memories of going to the Macdougal Street restaurant back in the days when I lived in Greenwich Village. The evening was made that much more enjoyable for Geoff because Joel drove us to the restaurant, avoiding the hassle of public transportation.

I was also grateful to our friend John Doumanian, who would arrive at our apartment on his bicycle with CDs of Geoff's favorite traditional jazz. He'd settle on the couch with Geoff to listen to music and tell me, "Go on, scram. Get outta here for a while." When I wanted to meet my agent for lunch or needed to do errands, I timed the outings to his visits.

Another source of fun and companionship was my pool of "Bunny" friends, the women I'd worked with at the Playboy Club when I was a student at the American Academy of Dramatic Arts back in the 1960s. Tia, who had become a celebrated bridal millinery designer, would cook elaborate Italian feasts in her spacious East Side brownstone for an ever-rotating guest list of former Bunnies, all of whom doted on Geoff. Occasionally we would all gather at Elaine's on the Upper East Side, our haunt since our Bunny days. As often as we could manage it, we would cadge a table at Rao's, the Harlem eatery run by Frankie "No" Pellegrino, once a room director at the Playboy Club and still loyal to his "girls."

One evening over dinner, Geoff said, "We ought to move here. It's so easy."

I laughed and had to agree. With good friends and so much to do, much of it within walking distance, New York living was indeed easy. We had only to take a crosstown bus to hear big band jazz at Birdland, or walk down to the end of our street to enjoy a cool breeze off the river. Best of all, Geoff had me entirely to himself.

However, the real purpose of our trip was the annual Dark Shadows Festival, a three-day event that Geoff looked forward to as much as I did. On a hot, muggy Friday morning in mid-August, a car picked us up to take us to a hotel in New Jersey, the venue for the 2009 festival. Some two thousand fans attended, many of them representing the generation who had "run home from school to watch" the ABC Gothic romance soap that featured vampire Barnabas Collins. But there were also younger fans who had grown up watching the 1,225 episodes in reruns or on VHS and DVD.

Jonathan Frid, the eighty-five-year-old actor who had portrayed Barnabas Collins, attended, as did Lara Parker, David Selby, Marie Wallace, Nancy Barrett, Jerry Lacy and many of the other actors I'd worked with on the series some forty-three years earlier. Everyone was so solicitous of Geoff, who sat in the audience while I was on stage for panel discussions and joined me afterward while I signed autographs.

The month in New York had been one of our most enjoyable stays, and Geoff was not at all happy about returning to Los Angeles. Our reentry into quotidian life without houseguests or another trip planned was not particularly smooth. Geoff looked longingly at the pool, but we both knew I couldn't manage to get him in and out by myself. Once again, he was left alone for an hour or so each day while I bought groceries and ran other errands. I packed pillows around him on the couch so he'd remain secure watching Turner Classic Movies until I returned.

I'd often come back to find pillows strewn all over the room because he was helpless to stop his hand from involuntarily picking them up and tossing them. I learned not to leave the remote control in his lap, because his fingers would clamp on the wrong buttons, increasing the volume to a deafening pitch or changing the channels in rapid succession. If he dropped the remote on the floor, he'd reach for it and slide off the couch. I couldn't leave him with snacks in case he choked. Each one of these scenarios raced through my mind during the hour I wasn't at home.

Somehow I managed to find time to write. My literary agent had good news for me, but it entailed reworking a manuscript she'd submitted. I was excited and eager to start rewriting, but it was clear I'd have to work around Geoff's needs. I ordered a Kindle and showed him how to press buttons with his thumb so he could read *The New York Times* and *The Wall Street Journal* on his own. I pulled a comfortable chair into my office so he could be near me while he read and I worked—not the best of all possible worlds, but the best I could come up with. Still, time and again he required assistance. He'd drop the device on the floor or lose his place, want food or drink, need to talk, ask to watch CNBC to check the stock market—it was endless, and I grew steadily more impatient with each interruption.

"You're rolling your eyes," Geoff would say. "Stop sighing."

The occasional forgetfulness that I had blithely referred to as typical male inattention had turned into more frequent bouts of confusion and disorientation. He often joked about "losing his marbles," but neither one of us wanted to think spells of befuddlement were signs his mind was slipping. Flip comments on my part were no longer funny and only drew attention to what we both feared might be symptoms of dementia.

One day, Geoff informed me that Princess Di had dropped in to visit him. I'd apparently missed her while I was in the kitchen preparing lunch. She didn't stay long, Geoff said, "but she'll be back." She continued to check in on him now and again, but her spectral visits seemed to coincide with my absences. He'd always had a soft spot for her and we'd stayed up to the wee hours of the morning to watch her funeral on television. I was glad she found time to drop in when she sensed he'd appreciate her company. "Next time, say hi from me," I would tell him. It seemed pointless to make an issue of it.

In terms of practical matters, Geoff did not want me to hire home help. Nor, frankly, did I after hearing about the home care problems Mari and Nancy dealt with. Geoff didn't want someone hovering over him. He preferred sitting on the leather couch in the den, watching cable news or vintage films, as long as I checked on him periodically. "Every twenty minutes would be good," he decided.

I gave him a cowbell to ring if he needed me. Unfortunately, if he dropped the bell and reached for it, I would find him on the floor. Worse, he would forget I'd told him I'd be gone for an hour and begin ringing the bell moments after I left the house. I'd return home, unlock the front door and hear a bell clanging. Geoff would be angry and worn out, shouting that he'd been ringing the bell "all day."

"You're not listening upstairs. Why couldn't you hear me?"

"Because I wasn't at home!"

"How was I supposed to know that? Just check every twenty minutes—and listen!"

I did "listen" to Geoff and I heard his frustration. It wasn't just that I couldn't hear him ringing the bell, but it was also his misery at being left alone to while away his days. He felt he had no purpose, that he was a burden. Even though we were together up to twenty-three hours a day, I was still too inaccessible. I'd cut out a lot of my outside activities, but I still had errands, household and business matters to deal with, besides trying to eke out time for my work. No wonder he'd concocted sporadic visits from Princess Di to keep him company!

Yet I couldn't allow Princess Di's clandestine visits to crowd our marriage, either. If he summoned her spectral presence to bring romance to his life, it was because it was slipping out of ours. I keenly felt the loss. While men may sometimes fall in love with their nurses, a wife assuming a caregiver role can spark the opposite reaction. Despite the moments of warmth and tenderness we still shared, marital intimacy of the sort we'd long enjoyed began fading with Geoff's physical deterioration and our changing roles. The sweet endearments vanished as he lost his voice. His touch was no longer so much one of longing as of a reach for safety and security. However, I still felt a thump of happiness when I caught a glint of mischief in his eyes, and I knew he still felt a wave of love for me when I held him close. With so much else changing in our lives, I couldn't bear to lose whatever vestiges we still had of the physical love and desire that had been such a valued part of our relationship. In a very conscious and purposeful way, I made time for intimacy between us.

I also realized that despite taking him to physical therapy and working with him on his exercises at home, I'd been taking Geoff's decline for granted since his shoulder surgery. That wasn't a healthy course for either of us.

I set about making some changes. Had Geoff not fallen and broken his shoulder, I would have followed up sooner on Dr. F's suggestion to consult with Dr. Yvette Bordelon. I called the Neurology Department at UCLA to book an appointment. Perhaps enrolling Geoff in a clinical drug trial would make him feel engaged and give him some hope.

Meanwhile, I cut down on my "busyness" so I had more time to just be with Geoff, to sit still, with my attention entirely on him. We had dropped out of UCLA's Plato Society. I'd also stopped working in the homeless program at my church, given up my seat on the board of the Beverly Hills Women's Club and decided not to take on any new publishing projects. I still managed to go on a few commercial auditions. When I was with Geoff, I made a conscious effort not to show any sign that caring for him was bothersome. If the phone rang while he was talking, I let it ring. If he dropped something on the floor, I picked it up without a sigh.

No one had to tell me that my brisk, busy-woman behavior was an attempt to avoid thinking about the inevitable. Sighing and rushing around kept me from bursting into tears. The heart of my problem was that for me there could be no "blissful denial." I dealt on a daily basis with the devastating reality that there was no treatment, no cure available for the man I loved and cherished. I had only to look at photographs of Geoff taken weeks before the fall to see what a massive setback the shoulder injury had proven to be.

There were times when I'd catch a glimpse of Geoff and see someone I barely recognized. A lump would rise in my throat. I had to either leave the room for a few minutes or somehow manage to mask my feelings. My mother hadn't wanted to see tears, and he most certainly didn't. The garden became my refuge. I'd smile, ruffle his hair and hold in the terrible surge of emotion until I could break away for a few minutes alone.

Participating in a clinical trial would help us both focus on something positive; if not a cure, perhaps a means of slowing the progression of his condition. Besides, Geoff was at his best engaging with people. He needed to feel there was still purpose to his life. He immediately brightened when I told him I'd called to book an appointment with Dr. Bordelon with the intention of getting him signed up as a "guinea pig."

Our initial appointment in early October 2009 was with Dr. Bordelon's husband, Dr. Carlos Portera-Cailliau, who was also associated with the movement disorders program in the Department of Neurology at UCLA. We arrived early for our ten a.m. meeting. As I reached into the back seat for the thick medical folder, Geoff asked, "Will you be gone long?"

"You're coming with me. We're here to see the doctor, remember?"

Geoff looked confused. "I thought you wanted me to wait in the car for you to come back."

"I think it's probably better if you come in with me," I said.

My tone was matter-of-fact, but my heart was sinking. We weren't off to a good start, but at least my response had been temperate. *Patience!* I helped him out of the car and we walked arm in arm into UCLA's Department of Neurology.

Dr. Portera, a slender, dark-haired man with expressive eyes and a gentle manner, immediately put Geoff at ease. I again refrained from speaking much during the session, although Geoff kept looking to me to answer Dr. Portera's questions. Geoff's once powerful and distinct voice had become more faint, and he responded using as few words as possible.

During the familiar battery of neurological tests, it was apparent his motor skills were rapidly diminishing. He had difficulty clapping his hands, tapping his foot, making a victory sign, miming opening a box or striking a match. He required assistance getting out of a chair and walking down the hall. His gait was reckless and inconsistent.

Dr. Portera agreed with the doctors from the Mayo Clinic and Columbia Presbyterian about increasing the carbidopa/levodopa dosage, but also thought it worthwhile trying Requip (ropinirole), a dopamine agonist, warning us that there was a potential for hallucinations and compulsive behaviors with the medication. (Would Princess Diana drop by more frequently?) He also recommended that Geoff consider using a walker or wheelchair to prevent falls. I told him we were already making occasional use of a transport chair, but I doubted Geoff had the necessary coordination to use a walker on his own.

Dr. Portera suggested that Geoff see Dr. C, an ophthalmologist, to determine if he might have PSP rather than CBD. "It's difficult to tell at this point, but I lean more toward a diagnosis of PSP."

As we were finishing our session with Dr. Portera, his wife, Dr. Bordelon, slipped into the room to join us. Following introductions, we chatted together for a few minutes about various clinical trials. Both doctors indicated that Geoff's general good health and motivation to participate were strong attributes in his favor for acceptance into a clinical study.

Heartened by this news, we followed Dr. Bordelon to her office on the other side of the reception area. The petite blonde had a gentle manner and was as soft-spoken as her husband. Geoff immediately warmed to her. More than that, he turned on the charm. I realized he'd gone into audition mode, hoping to dazzle her into accepting him into one of the programs.

Dr. Bordelon told us she was working with Dr. Irene Litvan at the University of Louisville on an observational study that did not provide treatment, but would also not limit Geoff's participation in a drug-testing program. While Geoff hadn't yet been officially diagnosed with PSP, Dr. Bordelon suggested Geoff might be a candidate for this observational PSP study, the purpose of which was to gain an understanding of genetic and environmental factors that might be associated with the disease. In this case, Geoff would need a "control," and I quickly agreed to join the study with him.

The second PSP study was for Noseiran, a Phase II

program for a drug with the protocol number NP031112 that might begin recruiting candidates as early as January 2010. According to Dr. Bordelon, Geoff appeared to be a good candidate for this program because he exhibited two definite signs (falling and eye palsy) and had no other underlying condition. UCSF was also working on a drug program study, but there was as yet no protocol number for it.

We set up a schedule of appointments for our individual screenings. Geoff also agreed to participate in another study that would involve periodic X-rays, blood tests and cognitive exams to record the advancing stages of his disorder—a guinea pig, indeed.

"Well, now we're getting somewhere," Geoff said as we left the clinic. If he could have tap-danced to the car like Gene Kelly, I think he would have. I was thrilled because it would mean that throughout the course of these clinical studies, Geoff would have the benefit of excellent medical care. I couldn't imagine a better team to have on our side than Dr. Portera and Dr. Bordelon.

Yet I also took to heart the warning of a young research assistant, who said, "Unfortunately, there's often great disappointment when someone doesn't fit the criteria for these testing programs and doesn't get accepted." I knew not making the team would be devastating for Geoff.

Within weeks, Geoff had appointments with two ophthalmologists, Dr. C and Dr. L. They both reported the same diagnosis: PSP, based on Geoff's clear inability to shift his eyes up and down, a hallmark of the disease.

Noting our schedule of appointments at UCLA, Geoff pointed out that we'd have plenty of time for travel in January. "How about a cruise?"

"Where do you want to go?"

"We haven't been to South America. I'd like to see Rio."

"Of course," I bantered. "I can just see us there celebrating Carnival!"

We both laughed, but I sensed Geoff was serious about taking the trip. A day or so later, he asked me if I had looked into a South American cruise. I told him I hadn't because I wasn't sure we were up to it.

"Really? I feel great. Besides, if not now, when?"

Indeed, those words had become our mantra. Clearly he wanted to go, so I went online and began checking cruise schedules.

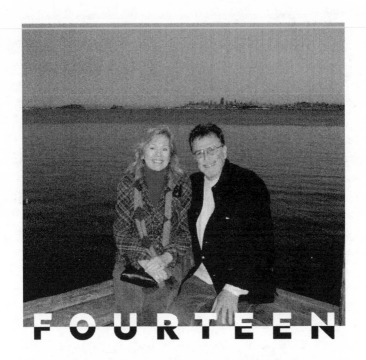

FOURTEEN

"LET'S GET AWAY
FROM IT ALL"

Thanksgiving 2009—We set out on our five-day trip up the coast in beautiful weather; crystal-clear skies, sunny and warm. We stay overnight in Morro Bay near the Hearst Castle at the Cavalier Oceanfront Resort, where the handicap rooms are state of the art; safe and beautifully designed. In the late afternoon, a short walk and picnic at a favorite spot with a view of the ocean ... and our traditional picnic bag packed with sausage, *cheese, bread, fruit and oatmeal cookies. We linger, watching the sunset, and return to our room just as darkness falls.*

We spend the evening sitting in armchairs in front of the fireplace, talking and listening to music. The following morning, I'm able to bathe and dress Geoff, give him his medications and let him relax in a comfortable chair looking out on the ocean while I take my time getting myself ready. The restaurant adjoining the inn has Geoff's favorite buckwheat pancakes and apple-smoked bacon. We're on the road by 9:30 a.m., arriving at the Ragged Point Inn just south of Big Sur a little over an hour later. Life is perfect.

In many ways our Thanksgiving trip in 2009 was far less fraught with anxiety for me and discomfort for Geoff. The beautiful weather was a bonus, although the previous year's woodsy picnic in a chill mist under a canopy of pine branches had its romance. But the major difference was that we were more knowledgeable about Geoff's condition and could therefore cope more easily with his limitations. He wasn't short-tempered, and I managed to curb my tendency to be impatient one minute, overly solicitous the next.

While Geoff rested, I scouted the rugged terrain for a suitable location for our treasured picnic. I found the perfect sunlit spot down a short path to a bluff above a cove with a spectacular view of the ocean. But even the brief walk was taxing for Geoff. After our leisurely picnic, we slowly made our way back to the room. While Geoff napped, I took a more adventurous walk.

By the time I returned from my hike along the headlands, Geoff was just waking up. I tucked a split of champagne and two glasses into a shoulder bag and, with the sun already low on the horizon, we strolled to a bench on the point overlooking the ocean.

While sipping champagne and watching the sunset, Geoff reminded me I should confirm our reservation for the cruise to South America in January before it was too late. I was well aware of the deadline. Although he had his heart set on taking a twenty-one day cruise from Valparaiso, Chile, to Rio de Janeiro, Brazil, I'd been uneasy about actually booking it. With two months to go before departure, I was concerned that he might not be mobile enough by then for me to manage on my own.

However, I took some comfort in my familiarity with the cruise ship. I knew the configuration of our stateroom and what I would need to bring to accommodate our needs. I also had confidence in their medical staff, because Geoff had received excellent care for an ailment on a previous cruise. But I was concerned about being so far from home if there was a big shift in his physical or mental state.

Yet it was also clear nothing would dissuade Geoff from going on the trip. As the sun blazed copper and magenta on the horizon, we chatted about the itinerary that would take us to Chile, Uruguay, Argentina and Brazil. The evening air grew cooler, but Geoff didn't want to go inside. He was enjoying the last glimmers of dusky daylight and the distant sounds of lapping waves. He asked for a warmer jacket and I hurried inside to get it.

When I returned only a minute later, Geoff was shaking with terror, certain that I'd abandoned him. I looked into his anxious eyes, trying to soothe him, and wondered how I could cope with moments such as these on a ship full of strangers, traveling far from home.

Two days later, Sunnie and Jackie picked us up in San Francisco for Thanksgiving dinner at the Buckeye, a wonderful restaurant in Sausalito. I'd been close to Sunnie since she was a teenager and worked part time for me in my publishing company. Now an accountant running her own business, she was happily married to Jackie, a lighting designer, and had moved to San Francisco.

Geoff's spirits were high, his humor so infectious that everyone, including the valet parker, responded warmly to him. Seeing that Geoff had difficulty getting out of the car, the valet offered us the use of a wheelchair for the steep incline to the restaurant. Geoff relished having Jackie push him up the slope, joking hilariously about the benefits of being an invalid. Dinner was delicious, and Geoff joined in the spirited conversation throughout the meal.

But the following morning, he awoke early and in a bad mood. He was agitated and immediately launched into a tirade about the Italians we'd had dinner with the night before, "who are trying to fleece us out of royalties on our cartoon films." What Italians? What cartoons? What royalties?

"Oh, I thought that was a business dinner," he said, when I questioned him. I reminded him we'd had dinner with Sunnie, who is Korean, and Jackie, who is Chinese, and there was no talk whatsoever about any film or cartoons, nor were there any Italians present.

"It must have been another night," he said, his rage undiminished.

He was still disgruntled as I checked us out of the hotel. By the time I'd loaded up the car and we were on our way, Geoff admitted he was probably mistaken about cartoon royalties and larcenous tablemates, but he was still grumpy. It occurred to me that Geoff had been looking forward to our annual trip and didn't want it to end. He needed something else to anticipate, if only as a distraction. He couldn't read. He could barely talk. His strength was sapped and he was aggravated by his physical limitations, and his mind was playing tricks on him.

I knew he'd also benefit from some steady companionship besides me. On the long drive home I suggested it was time to adopt a kitten to replace our beloved Maybelline, who'd died two years earlier.

Even on a holiday weekend, we found an animal shelter open in North Hollywood. Geoff took his time, cradling one furry bundle after another before settling on a sweet-faced tabby we named Daphne. Is there anything more enjoyably distracting than a kitten? He and Daphne bonded immediately.

I also booked our cruise to South America and acquired visas for Brazil. Dr. Bordelon assured me that we would not miss out on recruitment for either of two potential clinical drug trials, both in their last stages of gaining approval. The studies we'd signed up for were both worthwhile, but what we really wanted to do was enroll in a drug trial.

On December 8, we had a ten a.m. appointment to begin the observational PSP study, in which I was serving as Geoff's "control." In advance, we both had to fill out demographic and occupational history forms that would be used in the study to evaluate the genetic and environmental risk factors for PSP. We sat at the kitchen table filling in the required information, laughing that of the two of us I appeared to have the riskier background.

Geoff had grown up in affluent Brentwood and

Beverly Hills neighborhoods, spending most of his work-ing life in an office environment. Because my Norwe-gian father owned a farm in Norway, our family had been among the first wave of civilians permitted to travel by ship back to my father's homeland after World War II, where we lived while I was a toddler. When we returned from war-torn Norway to Minne-sota a year later, we lived on a farm where I was ex-posed to DDT and other pesticides. I'd lived and/or worked in England, Switzerland, Spain, France, Italy and Germany, and traveled extensively in Africa. What would their observational study make of all that?

Our days were filled with appointments in UCLA's Department of Neurology and the last of Geoff's physi-cal therapy sessions for his shoulder. He thrived on all the attention, especially if we followed a doctor's ap-pointment with lunch at the beach. Steve Randall, a writer and editor who had worked for Geoff at *Los An-geles* magazine, was one of our favorite lunch compan-ions at Chez Jay. We also managed to meet up with Jean, Lew, Warren, Burt, Nancy and other former col-leagues at the magazine, who were wonderful about staying in touch.

Keeping Geoff active and social made all the dif-ference in the world to his well-being, but it was a jug-gling act for me. In early December, I booked a commercial for a bank. Fortunately the filming fell on a Wednesday, coinciding with Candy's day to work at the house, so there was little disruption for Geoff. I also arranged for Gil and Miranda to stop by to visit him in the afternoon.

In case I had to hire someone for the day, I'd al-ready interviewed the manager of a home care agency.

The woman came highly recommended and was, in fact, an acquaintance of our housekeeper. The scowl on Geoff's face when the woman arrived for the interview told me that he still wasn't open to the idea of home care help.

I didn't want to impose too much on friends, nor overburden Candy. However, she made it clear that she was more than willing to help out—as she had done when Barbara was ill. As his condition declined, she pitched in without comment, giving him a hand up the stairs or helping him eat. She offered to make herself available if I needed someone to stay with him, but I was concerned about her safety if he fell against her small, five-foot frame. I repeatedly asked Geoff not to ask Candy to help him stand or walk, but he felt comfortable with her—and she was devoted to the man who'd helped make her family's life in the United States possible. But Candy and I both knew the time was coming when having a trained home care aide would be essential.

We planned to be in New York over the holidays, but the focus of the trip was filming interviews for a documentary based on my *Opera News* article, "The Star and the Stalker." Anne Pick, an Australian film director, and her husband, Canadian producer/director Bill Spahic, who run a film production company based in Toronto, had committed to producing a feature documentary about Nell Theobald, the former classmate of mine who had stalked Swedish opera singer Birgit Nilsson for nine years. We'd scheduled two days of filming in New York with my old friend, producer Stuart Goodman, who had secured permits for location filming on the streets of New York December 29 and 30.

My biggest concern was what to do with Geoff while I was filming for two days. I couldn't leave him alone for ten hours, and he'd made it clear he didn't want a "sitter." Naturally enough, Geoff wanted to be in the thick of it with us while we were filming. Stu solved the problem by renting a fifteen-passenger van for crew and equipment so Geoff could sit in the front seat watching while we worked.

Our good friend, the Welsh baritone Sir Thomas Allen, had agreed to do an on-camera interview on December 30, following his rehearsal for *Der Rosenkavalier* at the Metropolitan Opera. The night before we began filming, Geoff and I took Tom and his wife, Jeannie, for dinner at the National Arts Club, giving us a chance to catch up since we'd last been together in London. Geoff was full of entertaining stories he'd saved up to tell, and I didn't protest when he ordered a martini.

The following morning, I awakened very early so I could bathe, dress and feed Geoff before getting myself ready for a long day of filming. It was a relief knowing I wouldn't have to worry about him while I worked. Geoff loved being in the heart of the action, and Stu made him feel like part of the company by dubbing him "associate producer in charge of securing the van" while we were on location.

The weather was a frigid minus two degrees with severe wind chill, but Geoff remained toasty warm in the van. I was bundled in a warm coat, but my face was immobilized by the icy gusts. I could barely speak. We managed to film my walk-and-talk segments at several locations around Lincoln Center, then broke for lunch at PJ Clarke's. Afterward, we headed down to Wall Street for an interview with the attorney who had represented Nell in a personal injury lawsuit resulting from a freak attack by a lion she was posing with during a modeling shoot. At the end of a long, exhilarating day, Stu delivered us back to the apartment. I made a light dinner at home and we were in bed by nine o'clock.

The temperatures were milder the second day of location shooting on the East Side of Manhattan. By late afternoon we were back in our apartment recording some of my voiceovers. Tom Allen arrived for his on-camera interview to talk about the rigors of an opera singer's life and his own experiences with obsessive fans. Brian Kellow, one of the editors of *Opera News*, joined us for drinks with Tom and his wife after we wrapped for the day. I was feeling celebratory when we went with Brian for dinner at a neighborhood restaurant—not least because it had been such a treat for Geoff. But without the support of friends, we wouldn't have been able to cope. Once again, I realized how important it was to keep him engaged.

December 31, 2009—Geoff and I are communicating better as a result of all this togetherness. He struggles to speak, so every word is treasured. He doesn't lash out or brood. I'm more patient. When I do get exasperated or sharp with him, he knows that the stress of keeping him safe while assisting him is sometimes overwhelming. I slipped and almost fell while shampooing his hair and vented my frustration in a torrent of cursing that made him laugh.

"I know," he said. "And it will get worse." I felt so bad. What if I'd taken him down with me! Afterward, I sat on the couch with him and read a chapter aloud from Pops, *the terrific biography of Louis Armstrong by Terry Teachout that I gave Geoff for Christmas. We spent most of the afternoon sitting together. I'm grateful for this time we have. It's been a year of*

great change, and I'm fearful of what's ahead. Yet we'll handle it together and hope for the best.

We're going to South America . . . As Geoff says, "If not now, when?"

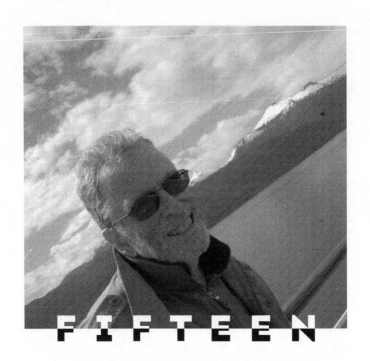

FIFTEEN

"SOUTH OF THE BORDER"

January 11, 2010—*I can't believe how well the "Star &
Stalker" shoot went! Or how well Geoff handled everything
from the long drive in the car to his patience while we were filming on the streets of San Francisco. Despite a tight schedule and
some tricky weather, everything came together. My two most
important interview subjects, who had both been reluctant to
appear on camera, were articulate, insightful and utterly credible.*

One man recalled events he hadn't mentioned when we first spoke two years ago, possibly because he's more trusting of me after seeing my article in print.

I also think he was more forthcoming after Geoff's quiet, encouraging chat with him while we were setting up the lights. Most astonishing, the man presented me with an envelope containing several original letters and documents from Nell that I could only hope existed. I did several standup pieces at other locations, including the San Francisco Opera House. Oddly, the trip turned out to be a trial run for the cruise because the rain and cool weather reminded me that "summer" well south of the equator might necessitate heavy sweaters and rain gear.

Also, the portable bath chair worked! I'm beginning to think we ought to stay in cheap old motels in San Francisco rather than swank hotels with quality handicap facilities. The roomy stall shower at the Wharf Inn was a dream. Geoff loved coming along on the shoot and I have peace of mind when he's with me. Also, we managed another delightful evening with Sunnie and Jackie—and this time Geoff didn't hallucinate about it afterward!

On the drive home from San Francisco, Geoff and I talked about the trip to South America. "Don't worry about me," he kept saying. "Just park me in a deck chair and go off on your own."

That option was neither realistic nor what I had in mind. I considered our cruise a pleasure trip that we would enjoy together. Considering Geoff's limitations, that meant preparing for every sort of contingency, both practical and medical. I spent hours going over our itinerary, checking online for weather conditions we might expect in each port. We had to be prepared for rain, both icy and tropical, and temperatures that could range from mid-forties to ninety-plus degrees. Instead of signing up for a tour package for port excursions, we decided to stay flexible and see what we could handle on a daily basis. Because I was familiar with the ship and our accommodations, I could visualize what was needed to safely and adequately take care of Geoff. I made copious lists, checking items off as I packed them.

I scouted the Internet and medical supply stores for weeks, searching for suitable equipment we might need on the cruise. I found a lightweight collapsible transport chair, weighing only twelve pounds, that we could take on board the aircraft. Geoff could still walk with my assistance, but for shore excursions and occasions when he felt fatigued he would need the transport chair. I also bought a lightweight collapsible commode/bath chair that folded up perfectly into one of the two pieces of checked luggage. I packed as much as I could in the recesses around the collapsible bath chair, but that still left little room for clothing for the two of us. Yet I knew that since I would be handling it all by myself, having too much luggage with us was as undesirable as having too little.

I remembered Geoff's comments years earlier about traveling with his first wife, Barbara, who required a wheelchair when her MS worsened. "People always seemed amazed we could have fun, that having a disability didn't have to be burdensome. If we looked like we were enjoying ourselves, people wanted to be around us." And with regard to Barbara, who took great care with her grooming, he said, "If you look nice, people treat you better."

But Geoff also treated me better when the bathing and dressing rituals went smoothly. I used the entire week before we left as dress rehearsal, enabling me to pack a grooming kit with exactly what we needed and clothing I knew I could get on and off him with a minimum of fuss. I even found warm, waterproof outerwear that looked enough like a safari jacket to keep him happy. He loved pockets.

Our single carry-on was stuffed with medications, medical supplies and anything we might need in case our luggage was lost or our flight delayed. As it turned out, weather and equipment delays on our flight to Santiago, Chile, utilized almost all my emergency supplies—extra disposable underwear, wipes, medication, antacids and chocolate. Geoff handled everything very well. We even managed a fairly dignified middle-of-the-night trip to the bathroom on the long flight out of Dallas/Fort Worth, if manhandling a six-foot man up an aisle and into a three-foot-square compartment can in any way be viewed as decorous. As we made our way back to our seats, Geoff was laughing so hard at my contortions inside the cubicle that I'm sure a few passengers wondered what we'd been up to.

I thought Geoff would want to collapse in bed as soon as we were aboard ship, but he was game for a white wine spritzer and light supper before we sailed. I was feeling celebratory because we'd made it on board without incident or injury—and the bath chair, fully assembled, fit perfectly in the shower stall! I crowed with delight as I ticked off my packing list and realized I'd left nothing behind. I was also grateful for the transport chair, which provided safe seating for Geoff while I dealt with immigration, baggage and a long trek to ground transportation.

Once safely in our room, I folded the transport chair and stored it in the closet for use on shore excursions. Our cabin was neat and orderly, showing no signs that the room was occupied by an invalid. I was determined to keep everything looking as normal as possible. Walking arm in arm, we strolled the upper deck, pausing at the railing to watch our ship pull away from the dock and sail into open water. Geoff, grinning like a school kid, was as happy as I'd ever seen him. "I wondered if we'd make it," he said, relief and exaltation evident as he squeezed my hand. The thought occurred to me that perhaps I should keep Geoff on one continuous cruise!

Our first day at sea was rough. Passengers feeling well enough to emerge from their cabins were clinging to railings and toppling against walls. Geoff joked that everyone looked in worse shape than he did. Neither of us felt queasy or suffered seasickness, but I played it safe, making sure a crewmember assisted me in getting Geoff in and out of chairs. As long as the sea remained rough, we had the dining rooms and decks virtually to ourselves.

On our third day at sea, we sat in the Horizon Room, with its unobstructed panoramic view, as our ship cruised through the fjords at the southernmost tip of Chile. In this land of midnight sun, we gazed at a pearl-pink sky illuminating snowcapped mountains, with a pale shroud of fog hugging the water.

In Puerto Montt, our first port, none of the shore excursions were suitable for Geoff, but he urged me to go ashore on my own. Geoff agreed to remain in the stateroom and not get up or move around while I was gone. I left him sitting up on the bed, pillows plumped around him, watching CNN. I was still queasy about leaving him alone, but felt better after arranging for a steward to look in on him regularly.

I disembarked midmorning, took the tender to the quay and walked through the small village. It was a beautiful sunny day, and the open market was brimming with colorful stalls stocked with fish, meat, cheeses and various prepared foods. I'm a farm girl, irresistibly drawn to displays of eggs, fruits and vegetables. I walked to the end of the quay, where packs of sleeping dogs were lying in the sun near fishing boats and then, unable to keep my worries at bay, hurried back to the ship.

When I returned, Geoff was napping but awakened as soon as I entered the cabin. He turned his head to me, his eyes anxious. I saw blood on the pillow and gasped. "It's nothing. Don't worry. I didn't fall."

I sat next to him on the bed, gently lifting his head from the pillow. The skin above his eye was scraped raw and there were scratches on his cheek. "Geoff, I'm so sorry, so sorry. I shouldn't have left. What happened?"

"Please don't say anything. Not your fault."

He was shaky and miserable. I felt so guilt-ridden I wanted to cry. Neither of us said anything for a long while. I gently cleaned his face with a damp cloth and applied antiseptic cream from my kit. The scratches weren't deep, but the skin looked burned, almost as though he'd rubbed it off. His body was warm, his face feverish. I held him close, calming him.

After a few minutes, he turned to me. "I need to talk to you," he said in a low, serious voice. "I was trying to reach for my eyeglasses, but my hand started to scratch my head. I couldn't stop. My hand does what it wants to. I put my glasses under the pillow and tried to sleep in order to stop."

I lifted the pillow and found his eyeglasses, one

stem slightly bent. "I'm so sorry. I should have stayed with you." I straightened the glasses and wiped blood from the lenses.

"It's just going to get worse. Can't help it. Not your fault. Not your fault. Not your fault."

Again, I held him close, feeling his anguish and trying to reassure him. Emotions for both of us were running deep. He knew how much I regretted leaving him alone. The anxious hour that he'd spent in pain, frightened that he was unable to stop scratching himself, was certainly not worth my walk through a market!

I sensed how bad Geoff felt, too, undoubtedly recalling his own years caring for Barbara and knowing how much I needed to have a little time to myself. The two of us sat on the edge of the bed, bound in misery, until Geoff said, "I'm hungry. Lunch?"

I laughed and the tears started to roll. How like Geoff! He gave me a wolfish grin. "I'm going to have a beer, too."

That morning's incident was remarkable in that it was a rare instance when Geoff recognized what he was experiencing and was able to describe it with insight and clarity. Most of the time he was oblivious to these involuntary actions and appeared hurt and bewildered when I intervened. He would look confused when I pushed a bowl of peanuts beyond his reach to stop him compulsively cramming handfuls into his mouth, which caused him to choke because he couldn't chew and swallow fast enough. I'd grasp his hand as he was about to involuntarily sweep something to the floor and he'd look at me with a puzzled expression. I grew used to his look of astonishment: *Now what?*

One of the most frustrating things about Geoff's

condition was recognizing each new phase as it developed. Even though we knew that one of the hallmarks of PSP was restricted eye movement and an inability to look down, it took me too long to realize how many everyday functions that affected. I chided him about tipping his head forward and looking at his feet when he walked. "That's why you're stumbling," I'd tell him, not understanding until he was diagnosed with PSP what his visual limitations were.

Sometimes he would close his eyes and look drowsy while he was eating. His eyes were constantly tearing up and he would wipe them with whatever was handy, occasionally a corner of a tablecloth, unaware that he was about to overturn his dinner plate. It took me way too long to realize he couldn't control his blinking. His eyes were dry and sore, causing him to scratch and rub them. He needed eye drops, not my constant admonishments to "please stay awake while we're eating!"

A big concern for me on the cruise was the chance Geoff would take another turn that I wouldn't immediately recognize or know how to handle. Most often a new phase began with some minor irksome behavior that was frustrating to both of us. So it was with Geoff's nonstop squirming on the third day of our voyage. He could *not* sit still. He sometimes squirmed to the point of tipping over a chair or sliding out of it. At first I thought his clothing was uncomfortable or he was signaling his need to go to the bathroom; neither was the case. We had gone through previous bouts of restlessness, but his requests to be "reseated" were near constant. My fierce looks and stern requests to "*please*, sit still!" were completely ineffective, only infuriating him

and frustrating me. Eventually the restlessness subsided, only to be replaced with constant thirst.

It didn't help that I was overly mindful of our behavior in public. Not knowing what sort of mood would
come over Geoff, I took every precaution to avoid
spoiling the enjoyment of other passengers or causing
ourselves embarrassment. I also didn't want to appear
to need too much assistance, although crew members
and other passengers readily gave me a hand holding
doors open or giving us wide berth in the narrow corridors. We dined early, sitting by ourselves at corner
tables where we could be private and not cause distraction. I cut up Geoff's food and assisted him with soup,
salad and other foods he could no longer eat by himself.

We quickly adapted to a morning routine that
avoided the bustle of other passengers assembling for
shore excursions. Our stateroom felt spacious, especially
with the large picture window and comfortable seating
area. I ordered breakfast from room service and then
spent a leisurely hour feeding, bathing, medicating, and
dressing him. I couldn't have managed without the
bath chair, especially when the sea was rough. While
he watched CNN, I bathed and dressed myself. Then
we'd stroll on the upper decks after other passengers
had disembarked.

Five days into our trip, all was well. Geoff's face
healed and his thirst subsided. He'd stopped demanding to be "reseated." He was thriving on the sea air,
walks, good food and my near-constant companionship.
We hadn't had to deal with constipation, diarrhea,
falls, choking, complications with medication or severe
mood swings, all the horrors I dreaded could occur. But
I remained cautious and alert, not wanting to attract the

attention of what I called the Hubris Dragon. The strain was sometimes intense and there would come a time almost every day when I had to get away and let the tears come—hard to manage on a cruise ship where privacy was at a premium.

Relief came in the form of various shipboard acquaintances occasionally joining us for cocktails and chats on deck. Geoff enjoyed the company of one man, in particular, and knowing they would be engaged talking for an hour or so enabled me to occasionally go off on my own. In fact, I secretly suspected this particular passenger of keeping Geoff company as a random act of kindness toward me. He would shoo me off with a wave of his hand and I would walk the decks on my own. How I loved the freedom of striding around the upper perimeter of the ship, arms swinging!

I checked daily to see how accessible the ports were. If the ship could dock and a tender wasn't necessary, we would disembark and use the transport chair to explore on our own. At the end of a quay there was often a car and driver available for private tour hire. I'd check out the car to see if the trunk would hold the transport chair, then chat with the driver to assess how accommodating he was and his fluency in English.

The only excursion I booked for myself was a catamaran trip to the glaciers in Laguna San Rafael on my birthday. Although it apparently rains thirteen out of fourteen days in that area, the weather was sunny and bright. After lunch, I seated Geoff in one of the lounge chairs in the Horizon Room, where his shipboard friend joined him for coffee. The men were pleased to have each other's company while I was on the tour. I set out on the two o'clock excursion to the San Valentin Glacier, confident Geoff was in good hands. I couldn't have asked for a better birthday gift than the relaxed, thoroughly enjoyable visit to the mammoth glassy blue icebergs.

When I returned, I discovered Geoff had asked one of the stewards to help him back to our stateroom. He was sitting in a chair watching a film on Turner Classic Movies, looking alert and pleased that he'd managed so well on his own. His spirits were buoyant as we dressed for dinner. He was so determined to make my day special and I loved him all the more for it. I knew it hurt Geoff that he had so little means left of showing his love. The husband who'd been so romantic and demonstrative in his affection for me could no longer surprise me with flowers or shop for the perfect little gift. He couldn't even rely on his voice or facial expressions to convey tender feelings, yet he'd managed to give of himself that day: the gift of being there for me.

The captain in the elegant Tuscany Room rearranged our corner table so I could sit facing the lagoon and assist Geoff eating. The scenery was magnificent: glassy fjords bordered by thick forest and snowcapped mountains glistened in the pearly pink evening sunlight. I ordered a good bottle of red wine and we enjoyed a leisurely dinner that concluded with chocolate birthday cake lit with candles. Afterward, we sat in the Horizon Room toasting the midnight sun with champagne. It was a day made perfect by Geoff's warm smiles and good spirits.

The following day we were on rough open sea with stormy rain and no visibility. Geoff was sleepy, distant and had such difficulty walking that we stayed in the room most of the morning. I was concerned because he was breathing through his mouth and his eyes had a dull, vacant look. He'd had only a small sip of wine, but perhaps even that had been too much. I read to him until he fell asleep, then curled up next to him and read my own book.

The warmth of his body next to mine was a comfort, filling me with tenderness, but with it an aching sadness. It was at times like these that I had to stop myself from thinking of a future without him. At least I was fit and healthy enough to make whatever time we had together as fulfilling as it could be.

One of our best days together was in Ushuaia, the southernmost port on the cruise. With the aid of four crewmembers, we hauled Geoff down the ramp and into his transport chair on the pier. By the time I pushed him to the end of the quay, I knew I wouldn't be able to negotiate the hills or narrow, uneven sidewalks. I was arranging to hire a car and driver for the day when Craig and Barbara, one of the couples we most enjoyed being with, asked if they could join us on the tour of the parkland. Our driver spoke excellent English and couldn't have been more accommodating. Geoff's transport chair fit easily into the trunk and off we went.

The rugged scenery in Tierra del Fuego National Park was breathtaking. The driver took us to remote beaches and roadside vantage points that couldn't accommodate tour buses. Several times Geoff was game to leave the transport chair behind in the car and walk with my support, which enabled us to navigate a stretch of beach and a spongy forest path to a beaver dam. I was gleeful that we were able to traverse a tricky walking bridge to reach a strip of land designated as the tip of the continent—Antarctica dead ahead across the Bering Sea!

Afterward, our driver dropped us off at a restaurant with a great view of the port and within walking distance of the ship. We shared a bottle of local wine with Craig and Barbara and enjoyed plates of delicious king crab.

In Port Stanley, the Falkland Islands, we managed to get Geoff and his transport chair aboard the tender, then up a steep ramp onto the pier. This time the two of us were on our own, and I realized almost immediately that I'd taken on too much. Slogging up hills and wrestling the small transport chair wheels over broken curbs was arduous. But the air was crisp, the sun warm as we traveled the length of oceanfront past Christ Church, Thatcher Drive and the war memorial to the governor's residence and back again. We somehow managed to avoid buying any penguin souvenirs, but couldn't resist pushing up the steep slope to the Globe pub so Geoff could enjoy a few sips of Guinness.

We were both exhausted by the time we were back aboard ship. We sat on deck chairs, Geoff napping while I read. When he awoke, his mood had shifted dramatically. The ship had sailed into open seas and begun rocking in the swells, unsettling him. He was irritable and scowling. He wanted to go back to our room. I asked a steward to assist me in getting Geoff to his feet and walking with us to the elevator. On the way, Geoff said he was hungry. I suggested stopping in the Terrace Café. If only I'd said nothing, taken him back and simply ordered room service!

To my deep regret, I missed all the signals that he had become disoriented. I'd only confused him by suggesting a change in plan. By the time we reached the elevator, the ship was rocking and pitching. Geoff was tense, showing signs of panic. The elevator door opened and the four people crowded inside urged us to get in. I told them we'd wait for the next elevator, but by then they'd moved aside to make room. The steward pushed us inside, and I knew the moment we stepped aboard that it was a mistake. Geoff was unable to grab a hand-rail in the crowded cubicle and became even more agitated.

The other passengers were in high spirits. One of them exclaimed, "What a glorious day!"

Geoff waved his hands and snarled, "Glorious! Glorious! Glorious!"

The other passengers realized immediately what was happening and tried to calm him, but Geoff kept shouting, "Glorious!" The moment the doors opened on the next floor, I edged Geoff out. One of the passengers held the door and asked, "Weren't you going up to the Terrace Café?"

"No, no," I said. "A little too bumpy for us."

Geoff stumbled against the wall, almost falling over, shouting at me, "Make up your mind, make up your mind, make up your mind!" as the elevator doors closed.

Several other passengers approached us in the hall-way as I tried to soothe Geoff and stabilize his footing. One of the men grasped Geoff's arm and helped me walk him back to our room. I thanked the man, closed the door and wrestled Geoff into a chair. By then he was shaking violently and I was sobbing.

"You can't do this! We're going to get kicked off the ship!"

"Good! They were being sarcastic."

"They were not! They were being friendly and kind!"

"Sorry. Sorry. Sorry. Can't help it. Can't help it. Can't help it."

"Yes, you can! You promised no outbursts, no public scenes. You can't blame it on your condition!"

"Sorry. Sorry. Sorry."

"Then don't do it, do it, do it, damn it!"

As soon as the words sprang from my mouth, I was sorry. I knew he couldn't help it. Rapid mood shifts and displays of agitation and anger were hallmarks of his condition. I was ashamed of myself for my own overreaction, but I couldn't help it, either, damn it!

I cringe when I see people vent anger in public. The prospect of being personally involved in a quarrel or angry outburst on the street or in a restaurant is horrifying to me. Yet I had to get a grip on handling these situations, because it was clear they would continue to occur. Meanwhile, Geoff sat mute, looking contrite. I dried my tears and asked if he was hungry.

"No. I want to go home."

I laughed in spite of myself. "So do I, but I'm afraid we're stuck here unless we swim."

Geoff's face softened. He smiled. "Then I guess I'm hungry."

I ordered room service and checked the Turner Classic Movies schedule. Once again, I reminded myself that our time together was too precious to squander. I had to rein in my own emotions, but my stomach was still in knots. I dreaded spending a sleepless night, my brain churning. Over and over I replayed my litany of errors, knowing it was my fault: Beer, sweets, a rocking ship and an overpeopled elevator were too much for Geoff. He needed down time.

Still. His outburst cut deeply into my fears of public humiliation. My raw emotions found refuge in a storehouse of marital slights, misunderstandings and unresolved issues from the distant past that roiled up in the dark hours of a long, sleepless night. *After all I was doing for him! How dare he! How could he do this to me?* I knew my thoughts were irrational, but I couldn't help it.

In the early hours of the morning, I lay awake listening to Geoff's gentle, breathy whiffle as he slept. When he awakened, he brushed his knee against mine and looked into my eyes. "Sorry, I couldn't help it. I thought you'd know it's compulsive and forgive me."

Of course I forgave him. I understood. Daylight and the gentle stroke of his hand quelled my rage, only to be replaced by feelings of sorrow that we couldn't be the way we were. And never would be again.

After weathering that emotional storm, we sailed into smoother waters for the remainder of our trip. With no more harrowing incidents or outbursts, Geoff and I enjoyed a wonderful time together. Most days we joined our shipboard friends, Barbara and Craig, in hiring a car and driver for an independent tour. We were lucky in finding excellent guides in Buenos Aires, where we watched tango dancing and dined in local restaurants. In Rio de Janeiro, we made it to the top of Sugarloaf, toured the city and strolled Copacabana.

Everyone, not just Craig and Barbara, showed us great kindness. But then almost everyone on board was coping with some sort of health condition, visibly apparent or not. At the ice cream counter one day, a man

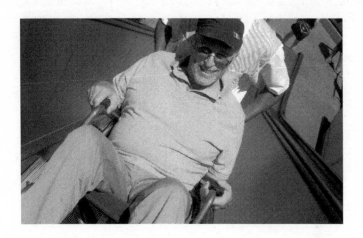

from Northern California asked me if I was traveling with my father.

The question startled me. How could anyone possibly think Geoff and I had a father/daughter relationship? Geoff was only a few years older than me—but then I glanced at him waiting at our table for me to bring him his sundae. He was slumped in his chair, his face expressionless, and I saw how much he'd aged. I told the man Geoff was my husband and that "we all age differently."

He agreed and added, "Especially after a stroke, I suppose." I explained that Geoff had a progressive neurological condition. He nodded toward his wife, a slim, very attractive blond woman seated nearby, also waiting for her ice cream. "She's had cancer for five years and is taking chemo even while on the cruise. Every day we have together is a gift."

To break our long return flight from Rio, we stopped in New York for a few days. I left some of the equipment I'd found so useful on the cruise behind in the apartment. Those few days gave Geoff time to decompress and get used to the idea that we were going home. He wanted to keep traveling.

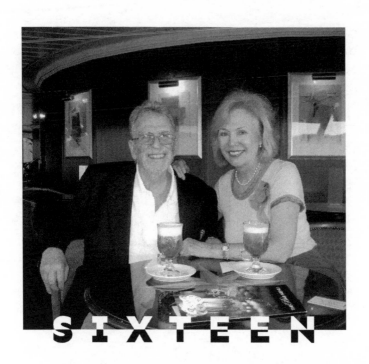

SIXTEEN

"LET A SMILE BE YOUR UMBRELLA"

Soon after our return from South America, Geoff turned another corner. He could no longer brush his teeth using the electric toothbrush, even when I switched it on for him. The toothbrush would fall from his hand. He could not wrap his fingers around a cup. His voice was weaker. He moved more slowly and sometimes stopped completely, unable to lift his feet until I gave him a little shove and urged him forward.

When I took him for short walks in the small pocket park at the bottom of Doheney Drive or the Will Rogers Memorial Park across from the Beverly Hills Hotel, we could no longer walk arm in arm. I had to keep a firm grip on his upper arm and support him with my other arm wrapped around his waist. He preferred not having me use a gait belt—a thick strap that buckled around his waist and gave me a secure grip—in public, so we managed without it. Getting him in and out of the car was a struggle because he was so stiff. I used my arms, knee, hip and shins to wedge him into the seat, then took a deep breath and struggled to attach his seat belt.

He suffered constant fatigue, drowsiness, sore eyes and cold hands and feet. He sat on his hands to keep them warm, and insisted I wrap him in a blanket even though he was wearing sweatpants, a thick sweater and the sheepskin-lined suede mittens that my sister-in-law had mailed from Minnesota. I had to feed him because he couldn't bear to take his hands out of the mittens. He no longer wanted a spritzer, the cocktail he'd looked forward to having while watching the evening news. The man who loved a good martini no longer desired any alcohol at all. He was listless, reluctant or unable to have any sort of conversation with me. In this condition, I would never have been able to care for him on the cruise as I had only weeks earlier.

Unfortunately, this change in Geoff's condition coincided with a flurry of jobs for me. I did two days of voice recordings and booked two on-camera commercials filming a week apart. The actors I worked with on the CD recordings were old *Dark Shadows* colleagues, so it was an easy matter to bring Geoff to the studio with me.

However, I was also gone for auditions and wardrobe fittings in addition to the long days spent filming on location, time that Geoff had to remain at home without me. There were early makeup calls and I had no idea when I might wrap for the day. I was thrilled about the work but stressed about arranging home care. Again I relied on Candy and friends to help out, but I'd also hired a home care aide. Geoff was not happy. He did not want a stranger assisting him to the bathroom or feeding him the meals I'd prepared. He would sit in sullen silence until I returned home.

Our world diminished. Geoff declined to use the transport chair when we went out. He didn't want friends to see him in it and think "the old buzzard's really going downhill."

We stopped going to weekend screenings at the Motion Picture Academy because it involved walking down a sloping aisle to a seat he had difficulty getting in and out of. Dining regularly in restaurants no longer appealed to him. Even with handicap facilities available, venturing out anywhere became cumbersome and too exhausting for him.

However, there were special events Geoff didn't want to miss, including a special screening of an early Noël Coward film at the Academy's smaller theatre in Hollywood. I remembered that the theatre had good handicap facilities and arranged for tickets. But even though we arrived early, we barely managed to get the last handicap parking slot. The walk to the theatre was longer than I remembered, and the screening room itself could only be reached using steep ramps and an elevator.

We took aisle seats in the back, but our row filled

with people who had to climb over Geoff, which made him grumpy. After the screening, people lingered in the aisles to talk. Geoff became impatient as we inched our way around clots of stragglers to the small elevator. On the way down to the ground floor, I asked him how he was feeling. "Hungry. I want pizza."

He was edgy, pale and very unsteady. He could barely stand, but we still had a long walk to the parking lot. We were almost there when I saw that a large van had parked too close to our car, leaving me no way to open the passenger door. Fortunately a young man hurried toward us to offer help. I leaned Geoff against the van, asked the young man to hold him up, and raced to pull the car out of the parking space. Even with assistance, it was difficult to get Geoff into the front seat. By the time I thanked the Good Samaritan and climbed back in the car, I was shaking so much I sat gripping the steering wheel until I was calm enough to turn on the ignition.

"How're you doing?" I asked.

"Hungry."

"Okay. I'm sure I have something at home."

"Pizza!" Geoff shouted. "Pizza! Pizza!"

I stopped for pizza, leaving Geoff in the car while I placed the order, then sat with him until it was ready. When we arrived home, I took a deep breath. We were safe. No mishaps, embarrassing incidents or trips to an emergency room. We enjoyed the pizza and talked about the movie. As I fed him the last of the pizza he put his hand on mine and said, "We should do this more often."

Two weeks later, on Easter eve, I took Geoff to a choral service at church. Midway through the service,

Geoff slumped in his seat and looked pale. I signaled an usher standing nearby, who helped me walk Geoff out of the church. Before we could reach the car, Geoff collapsed against me and slid from my arms to the ground. He wasn't unconscious, but he looked dazed. I propped him in a sitting position and braced him against my legs while deciding whether to call paramedics or try to take him home.

Within moments, I heard a siren and realized one of the ushers had already placed a 911 call. I was relieved the decision was out of my hands. Geoff's skin was clammy, his breathing shallow. The paramedics checked him out and insisted he go to hospital for tests and observation. It was the prudent choice, but I groaned—not Cedars-Sinai on the Saturday night of a long holiday weekend! I climbed into my Prius and followed the ambulance, reminding myself to always pack a book in my shoulder bag no matter where we went.

Keeping up a balancing act was hard on a constantly shifting tightrope. Yet I was determined to keep doing whatever we could to enjoy our lives together, whatever the consequences. When things went wrong, I'd just have to deal with it, including the inevitable bouts of tears and self-recrimination. I wondered: Will tomorrow be the morning I wake up and have a highball for breakfast?

In fact, one morning, I accidentally swallowed a cocktail of Geoff's medication. Groggy from a restless night, I was performing my early morning rituals on autopilot and somehow tossed his pills into my mouth instead of my vitamins. I realized my mistake as I swallowed.

For once, Geoff was more alert than me. "Aren't those mine?"

I smiled weakly. "Sorry."

"It's gonna make you sick."

"I hope so. If it makes me feel better, I'll be worried."

In spite of the jolly banter, my mind was reeling. *What the hell have I done to myself?* I tried not to think of the potential damage making its way down my esophagus, but I had little choice since Geoff still needed his medication. I reopened the array of bottles and tapped out another handful of carbidopa/levodopa, mirtazapine, omeprazole, Requip and allopurinol.

I reasoned that if this heady mixture hadn't killed Geoff, it wasn't likely to finish me off. My bravado lasted until I'd medicated Geoff, taken care of his other needs and settled him into a chair to watch CNBC.

Then I shakily made my way to the telephone to call the twenty-four-hour pharmacy. It was barely seven a.m., but someone answered the phone almost immediately. I explained that I had accidentally swallowed my husband's medication and listed the pills.

"What do I need to do? Go to emergency? Have my stomach pumped?"

"Wait, you did what? Why would you do that?"

"I know. A stupid mistake. Just tell me, is it serious?"

"If you're asking me, lady, I think you're gonna be real sick. You gotta be more careful."

It hadn't occurred to me that the person in the drugstore who answered my call might have been interrupted sweeping the floor or filling the candy rack. But pharmacist or not, the man was entirely correct. I barely had time to hang up and race to the bathroom before I was violently ill. No one has ever thrown up more joyously! I heaved in exaltation that I was up-chucking large bits of blue- and tangerine-colored pills.

When I'd finally emptied my stomach, I sat down on the edge of the bed, feeling oddly loopy, like a balloon sailing around, slowly losing air.

"Now you know how I feel," Geoff said.

"But you've built up a tolerance. Besides, I don't have gout or acid reflux." There was no need spell things out any further.

"You look pretty awful." He eyed me with what I mistook for sympathy and added, "How about some breakfast? I could go for buckwheat pancakes."

We were keeping to a regular schedule of appointments with UCLA's neurology department, but there was still no start date for enrollment in a clinical drug trial. My concern was that by the time the drug trials finally be-gan, the deterioration in Geoff's health would make him ineligible to participate.

It wasn't so much that we put on an act, but we were both on best behavior when we showed up for the appointments. I took care with Geoff's grooming and tried not to fluster him by rushing. I kept treats in my pocket to distract him if he became grumpy—it took little to set him off. I countered any brief spells of petulance by being overly bright and cheerful. I tried to find a parking space as close to the elevators as possible so we could leave the transport chair in the car and the doctors would see him on his feet, still managing to walk.

When he was having his periodic interviews or

cognitive tests, I stayed out of the examining room, hovering in the hallway like an anxious parent praying my kid would pass his entrance exams. On the way to the clinic, I'd often run through a quick drill so Geoff would remember the day of the week, his birth date, our street address and the name of the president of the United States. Just as often, Geoff would ask me questions so he'd have ready answers for a quiz. "Gotta keep the marbles rolling," he'd say, and we'd both laugh. It was clear that Geoff, too, wanted to make a good impression so he'd remain an eligible guinea pig.

Again, with assurances that we wouldn't miss out on enrollment for a clinical drug program, Geoff and I booked airline tickets for a six-week stay in New York. I impressed on Dr. Bordelon that we would return immediately if she sent word a drug trial was starting up. We did not want to miss our chance. The possibility that some as-yet-unproven medication would cure Geoff's disease was as remote as winning the Publishers Clearing House sweepstakes, but figuratively speaking we were perpetually all dressed up and waiting for Ed McMahon's life-changing knock on the door. We needed hope.

June 2, 2010—*I've tried to walk Geoff down the street and back for exercise, but he's shaky. Therefore, his muscle tone deteriorates even more. We've had some rough nights when I was up at least five times helping him rearrange his body in bed or get him to the bathroom. I lost my temper twice out of sheer frustration and then went overboard trying to make up for it. There are times when I'm so frightened and it comes out in anger. "Damn it, move!" I snarled, when he froze in the middle of the room on the way to the bathroom. What do I do when we are both half-naked and it's 3 a.m. and I can't get him to budge?*

It's especially difficult because he's so stiff. His strength is amazing. Trying to help him sit, stand, roll on his side in bed is almost impossible. I struggle, wrestling him around, trying to fight the resistance. He gets anxious and can't sleep unless I have my hand on his shoulder or back. My greatest fear is that we will lose communication and I won't even know what he wants or how I can help him. Then what? He looks frail, withered. He can't blow his nose. His eyesight is getting worse. The deterioration is terrible and coming on so fast now.

Without telling Geoff, I'd begun to turn down certain invitations. It was no longer fair to subject him or our friends to social gatherings that he just couldn't handle. I felt especially bad declining an invitation to a birthday celebration with Ann and John in their beautiful apartment overlooking Central Park. We loved their friends, and the food and wine were always sensational, but that sort of gathering with so many people was no longer appropriate for us.

But dinner with Hannah and Joel at Minetta Tavern to celebrate our nineteenth wedding anniversary was wonderful. They drove in from Connecticut, so we had their car to take us downtown and Joel's strong arms to walk Geoff into the restaurant. Hannah picked up his fork and fed him, taking over from me, and he loved her for it, flirting outrageously between mouthfuls. Afterward, we went back to the apartment for cupcakes and ice cream.

We managed to get to Birdland, too, sitting at our favorite ringside table. To celebrate Artie Shaw's 100th birthday, we went to a concert of his music, drank champagne and shed a few tears. Artie had been a close friend until his death in 2004. Geoff recalled that when pianist Joe Bushkin died, Artie had said he couldn't imagine living in a world without Joey. In turn, Geoff said, "Imagine, we're somehow living in a world without Artie."

One night, we went to the National Arts Club for dinner and to attend a staged reading of a Robert Anderson play with Frances Sternhagen. What a treat! As a bonus, we also discovered that there was a second elevator in the rear of the building that wasn't nearly as small and rickety as the one we usually used to get to the dining room. Those evenings were all very special, but we also spent many days alone together in the apartment. As often as we could manage, we'd go to one of the neighborhood restaurants in the evening.

One morning, our doorman mentioned that a neighbor had inquired about our bicycles in the basement storage room. The man had two children and wondered if we were interested in selling the bikes. I'd forgotten about the bicycles, which Geoff and I rode every summer we were in New York. One of our favorite pastimes was riding along the East River, then crossing into Central Park for a picnic. I went to the basement to check on them. The tires were flat, but they were in otherwise good condition. I remembered that the last time Geoff and I had taken them out was almost exactly two years earlier, when we'd bicycled through Central Park.

It was the same summer when my nephew Tom and his wife, Barb, sailed to New York from Newport, Rhode Island. We'd stood at the end of our street watching the two of them sail past us on the East River, then taken the subway to meet them at Chelsea Piers on the Hudson River. The four of us had spent a glorious time sailing around the harbor area and the Statue of

Liberty. Geoff's cherished Italian schoolboy cap had blown into the water and Tom had skillfully performed a "man overboard" maneuver to retrieve it.

Had we really managed those outings only two summers earlier? It seemed impossible. I told the door-man to please give the bicycles and helmets to the two youngsters in our building.

On the morning of June 2, I was packed and ready for the car to arrive a few hours later to take us to the airport for our flight back to Los Angeles. But I was also very concerned about Geoff, who seemed anxious and agitated. I became alarmed when I saw that he'd thrown up. His eyes were unfocused and he was pale. I was going to postpone our trip and call a doctor, but Geoff insisted he would be fine.

"Pancakes! Pancakes! Pancakes!"

"But you threw up! You want pancakes? Now?"

Geoff was adamant. I changed his shirt, wheeled him down the street to the coffee shop and ordered a short stack with a side of bacon. He ate it all and looked fully restored. I finished my coffee, wishing it could always be so easy to turn things around.

By the time we returned to the apartment, the car had arrived. Geoff was in good spirits, but I felt drained and still had to deal with airport security and a seven-hour flight. I had no idea what had caused Geoff's nausea or agitation, but perhaps both were brought on by anxiety over the flight home. In any case, I couldn't rely on the comfort of pancakes to see us through these occasions. I would have to ask Dr. Portera for some sort of "calming" medication to have on hand for Geoff's bouts of anxiety.

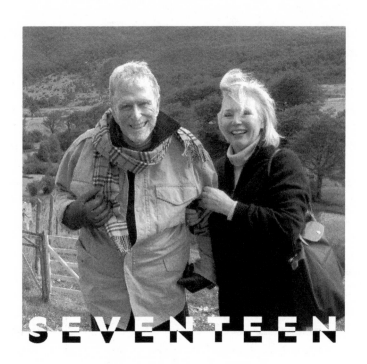

SEVENTEEN

"I HAD THE CRAZIEST DREAM"

Although Geoff was less mobile than he'd been on our cruise to South America, he wanted to be on the move again. He began planning another big trip, this time to the Caribbean, while at the same time showing little interest in going to restaurants or screenings in Los Angeles. He didn't want to deal with the everyday hassle involved in going out, very real reminders of his deteriorating health, but it didn't stop him dreaming about exotic travel and distant places.

But even as I was encouraging Geoff's enthusiasm to "hit the road again," I was also dealing with my dread of the next major "thing" that would slow him down even more. It was inevitable, so what fresh hell would we face? I recognized the pattern: There was always a plateau, a span of time when we managed to adjust to certain limitations before a sudden plummet to a new level of debility. Whatever it would be, it would happen without warning. I just hoped we could stave off another abrupt decline until after Geoff was accepted into a clinical drug program.

After a flurry of appointments at UCLA, we were both on tenterhooks about the possible new drug trial sponsored by Noscira S.A. in Madrid, Spain, that seemed tantalizingly close to starting up. We filled out more forms and remained hopeful.

Meanwhile, I cooked dinners at home, inviting one or two friends at a time to join us. Within minutes of finishing his meal, Geoff would signal that he was ready for bed. I would get him into the stair lift and our guests would wave him off as he made his slow ascent to the bedroom. He'd laugh and wave back, appreciating the lighthearted sendoff, but he would invariably tell me as I was putting him to bed that "it hurts to talk." At first I misunderstood and thought he meant it hurt not to be able to fully join in on a lively conversation. But the fact was that he suffered real physical discomfort trying to speak.

Cousins from Norway stayed with us for a week, followed by Jo-an and Adrian, our good friends from London. Thanks to strong, helping hands, we managed to get Geoff into the garden for long lunches and pool-side conversations.

Then, one day, I made another of my quick calls to a research assistant in UCLA's Department of Neurology to ask about the progress of the clinical drug trial. "Oh, yes," she said. "It's going ahead. We're already enrolling."

"What? But, but, but . . . " I sputtered. "Are we in? No one notified us. Is it too late?"

Eventually, after continued prodding on my part, Geoff was accepted into the double-blind, placebo-controlled Phase II study, and we were given an appointment for his first dose. If I hadn't made that routine call to that assistant, would we have missed that small window for enrollment? Also, had I not asked that research assistant specific questions about procedures, I would not have known that Geoff should fast before the appointment. Had he not fasted, he wouldn't have been given the medication and would probably have been eliminated from the program. I decided henceforth to err on the side of being a pest. When in doubt, I picked up the phone.

The initial session followed the usual protocol for our appointments in the neurology department. Geoff had to provide a urine sample, take an EKG, be weighed and answer a few questions—all relatively routine procedures unless you have PSP. Providing the urine sample meant wheeling Geoff to the toilet, which meant some inventive maneuvering on my part once we were in the stall and then threats and cajoling. He was simply not able to pee on cue. On one occasion I heard myself say, "Okay, no pee, no enchiladas for lunch!"

Taking his blood pressure, weighing him and getting him to lie still for the placement of the EKG sensor pads was difficult and continued to be more taxing with each consecutive appointment. I suspected that we had made it into the trial just under the wire.

At the end of the session, Geoff consumed his first dose of NP031112, a packet of powder mixed in a carefully measured portion of water. I watched closely, knowing I would be in charge of administering this medication at home. No one, including Dr. Bordelon, had any way of knowing if the dose was full strength, half strength or a placebo. Afterward, we carried home our precious cargo, two boxes of individual packets of powder that we dubbed "magic potion" and stored them in the refrigerator.

We were so thrilled that Geoff was in the clinical trial that we announced the news to everyone. We'd been told not to anticipate any great improvement, but we couldn't help looking for some sign that Geoff was getting better. At first we imagined that his voice was stronger, that he moved more easily. In fact, he was getting stiffer, less mobile, and we seemed to be sinking to a new plateau. He had so little control over his movement that unless I barricaded him with pillows, he would squirm off the couch and slide onto the floor.

Most days, I sat next to Geoff on the couch, doing rewrites on my laptop while he watched Turner Classic Movies or one of the financial news shows on cable. Now and then I would glance at Geoff sitting slack-jawed, his hands in thick mittens, staring fixedly at the television screen, knowing I was losing him day by day. He barely spoke unless he wanted something or needed assistance.

Somehow I managed to concentrate on my work

despite interruptions. Even when Geoff called me to "reseat" him when he was slipping down on the couch, wanted to change channels, needed something to drink or had to go to the bathroom, I was able to stay focused and return to my writing.

Then, one Tuesday afternoon at three p.m., I turned to Geoff and said, "Guess what? I'm done. My book is finished."

"Good. Read it to me."

I turned off the television and began reading aloud from *Dark Passages*, the paranormal mystery I'd written with a humorous wink and nod to *Dark Shadows*. Over the years, I'd written several nonfiction books about what really happened behind the scenes during my four years on the series. With *Dark Passages*, it had been fun to imagine what might have occurred had the ingénue lead been a real vampire.

It was a lighthearted story about a farm girl named Meg, who arrives in New York to fulfill her dreams of becoming an actress while trying to conceal her secret identity as a real-life vampire. Meg's mother, who is also a vampire, has provided her daughter with no training in how to exercise her considerable paranormal gifts or conduct herself in a world of mortals.

When I finished reading and asked Geoff what he thought, he said, "You know, you've written about your mother." I laughed, then realized that I'd indeed been unconsciously channeling her in writing about a relationship between mother-daughter vampires. What would she have made of that!

I was pleased to send the manuscript off to my agent in New York, but I also experienced a huge letdown. *Now what?* Writing a funny story about a soap opera vampire had provided distraction and emotional escape. I could flip open my laptop and enter a world of my imagination. With the work finished, I felt empty and depressed for days afterward. Frankly, it had become hard for me to face anything reaching an end.

Days later, my theatrical agent called with a last-minute audition for an automobile commercial, and the following day, I had another last-minute audition for a credit card commercial. In the end, I booked both jobs, two very lucrative national commercials. The scripts were humorous and the directors top-notch. But as thrilled as I was to get the work, I was also concerned about Geoff's care while I was filming.

He seemed to like Marisol, a slim young woman from the home care agency who looked after him while I went for callbacks and wardrobe fittings. But she'd only worked four-hour shifts and I was apprehensive about her ability to look after him for an extended period if I had early calls and worked late. She didn't seem very experienced or look strong enough to maneuver Geoff. I watched her using the gait belt and she appeared capable enough, but I had doubts. However, Geoff enjoyed her company and his cooperation was critical, so I booked her. I set out meals and snacks and went over instructions in case of emergency, and hoped for the best.

While sitting in a makeup chair on location, Marisol called my cell phone twice: The first call was to relay a request from Geoff asking where the chocolates were hidden; the second to ask if there were any cookies. Clearly Geoff had got the upper hand! Filming went well and I wrapped early. As I was leaving, I grabbed some cookies from the craft services table and raced home.

I'd only been gone for eight hours, but Geoff looked anxious when I arrived. He wanted me to take him to the bathroom. After sending Marisol home, I asked him what he thought of her. He smiled and said, "She's great. Have her come again."

I then discovered that he hadn't been to the bathroom all day because he didn't want to ask her to take him. Somehow I had to impress on him that she was a caregiver not a "date."

Four days later, I got the schedule for the two-day shoot on the commercial for the credit card company, which would be filming on location some thirty-five miles from home. To complicate matters, the first day of filming coincided with Geoff's appointment at UCLA for his two-week drug trial checkup. Thank God I could call on Harry! He agreed to drive Geoff and Marisol to the appointment and then bring them back home afterward.

I impressed upon Geoff that Marisol was there as a caregiver, not just to provide him with cookies and chocolate. I prepared a meal that I knew Geoff would like and left written instructions. All went well on the first day, largely because Geoff felt secure with Harry on hand and I was home relatively early.

On the second day, we filmed from early morning until late at night, shooting a howling blizzard in 104-degree temperatures at Ontario airport. It was an incredible scene with tall cranes, huge fans and mammoth trucks spewing ice, wind and soap bubbles at me— indeed, I felt like I was in Alaska during a fierce blizzard, rather than on an abandoned airstrip in a California desert. We wrapped well after ten o'clock that night and I didn't get home until past midnight.

Because I knew I'd be gone for up to sixteen hours, I'd arranged for Harry to stop by in the afternoon, and for Gil and Miranda to visit in the evening. They brought dessert and watched a film with Geoff. But when I got home, Marisol was sitting alone with him. He had not gone to the bathroom and refused to let her put him to bed. He was anxious and moody. He wouldn't look at me, and I knew he felt abandoned.

"When are we going to New York?" he whispered as I tucked him into bed.

September 2, 2010—I've just called to wish Aunty Pat a happy 94th birthday. She sounds great, loves to play cards and still misses driving her car. I've also sent emails to Ben's friends reminding them to send greetings to him for his 80th birthday. Chances are he'll spend his big birthday in a Palm Beach art gallery mounting an exhibition of his photography—a fitting beginning to another decade of creative work. He's just closed an exhibit at a gallery in North Carolina. How differently people age!

Geoff's world—and mine—became increasingly diminished, although life together was not without pleasure and spontaneity. I treasured our moments of playfulness, intimacy and tenderness, when we connected to the romance that drew us together in the first place. A wave of longing would wash over me, reminding me how precious our love for each other still was.

One evening while I was chopping vegetables to make soup, Geoff sat exercising using a simple pulley assembly that I'd hung over the kitchen door. Meanwhile,

Daphne, no longer a timid kitten, playfully batted her paws on the dangling cords, making us both laugh.

To give Geoff some exercise after dinner, I walked him up and down the hallway, both of us singing "Some Enchanted Evening" and "Bicycle Built for Two" to keep his pace steady. We'd discovered that singing released whatever lock in his brain caused him to freeze and prevented him from moving. But this time it was the phone ringing that interrupted our stroll. The caller turned out to be an event organizer inviting me to be a guest celebrity at a three-day fan convention in Nashville, Tennessee, later that month. I turned to Geoff and asked, "You want to go to Nashville?"

His face lit up. "Sure! Never been there."

I readily accepted because the invitation had come through a college professor we'd met at various *Dark Shadows* festivals, who was familiar with Geoff's condition. He offered to pick us up at the airport and promised a tour of Nashville. We knew we'd be in safe hands. The morning of our flight, I loaded our stash of "miracle potion" packets into a small cooler with ice packets and, as always, Harry drove us to the airport. We traveled with the transport chair and, this time, breezed through security.

During the two-day event, when I wasn't doing a panel discussion or signing autographs, Jeff, an author and professor who lived in Tennessee, took us sightseeing and to local restaurants known for their grits, greens and gravy biscuits.

Geoff insisted I also book a flight to New York as part of this trip so we could take full advantage of the week we had available before our next mandatory appointment at UCLA. In New York, we packed in Birdland, a Sidney Bechet concert, dinner with my nephew Tom and his wife, and lunch with my literary agent. Geoff was in great form throughout the trip, but I sensed we were due for another rough patch when we returned to Los Angeles. A "new normal" was upon us almost immediately.

September 28—*It's been a rough day or so since our return from New York. Geoff is barely able to walk. I've had a few frightening moments when I'm supporting him with the gait belt and he can't move. We sing. I knock his leg. I bump him from behind, but he stands frozen. This morning, I managed to get him into the stair chair, then had to run to the garage to get the transport chair out of the trunk of the car and set it up at the foot of the stairs. He likes to operate the control button on the stair chair himself, but this time he couldn't manage the steady pressure. With fits and starts, he made it midway down the stairs before I took over. I had considerable difficulty transferring him from the stair chair to the transport chair.*

I was shaken by the suddenness of the change in him and just not prepared for it. His voice is barely a whisper. I have to lean close to hear him. We're also dealing with occasional incontinence. I knew it would eventually happen, yet it's presented us with another, rather sudden "new normal."

October 5—*My biggest problem is coping with sleepless nights. I awaken four or fives times a night because Geoff is thrashing around caught in the sheets, needs to be covered or uncovered or have his face turned on the pillow. Even after I help him adjust, he spends another hour squirming and thrashing. I also have to take him to the bathroom multiple times a night. It means cinching the belt around him, walking him from the bed to the bathroom with both of us singing (!).*

It's always another struggle helping him at the toilet. With my chin tucked around an arm, a hip pressed to his thigh and one knee jammed against the wall, I somehow keep him balanced. His body locks and his grip on the safety bar is iron-tight, so it's all I can do to wrangle him down while at the same time supporting him so he doesn't crash onto the seat. It's a wrestling match between 180 pounds of unstable, steel-like strength against 125 pounds of careful leveraging and agility. After I've climbed back into bed, my limbs are shaking. I rarely get back to sleep before I hear his faint voice asking me to cover him or move his arm onto the pillow.

I try so hard not to get exasperated or angry. But sometimes fear and fatigue get the best of me. I'm constantly thinking ahead. I never move unless Geoff and I are fully clothed and I have planned all my maneuvers. If he falls on the floor or on top of me, we face disaster. I feel like I am constantly apologizing or explaining or cajoling. I seem to spend most of my time saying, "What?" The rest of the time I'm saying, "Sorry."

I'm tired. My time away from the house is carefully planned, but I'm nervous every time I venture out. A couple of friends have asked if they can help me by shopping for groceries or doing errands. Yet grocery shopping is a treat for me, one of my few justifiable chances to get out!

I try to write, but can only eke out the solitary time to do so when I've finished all my chores. Bathing, dressing, medicating and feeding Geoff takes an hour and a half every morning. Then I help him check all his stock market balances and assist him making trades. That's it.

Showering Geoff is tricky now, but as long as I can get him to walk and hold on to the grab bars, I can get him into the shower and safely seated on the bathing bench. Cleaning ears, clipping nails, trimming his beard and brushing his teeth take place in the shower, either before or after I've bathed him. The job I hate most is getting his socks on him!

October 9, 2010—I woke up crying. I'm exhausted. I

know I will hire help when caring for Geoff on my own becomes a safety issue. He's so adamant about not having a "stranger in the house," I almost feel home care assistance will hinder more than help. Or maybe the time to hire help is the day I really do have a highball for breakfast!

In fact, it was the following day that I hired Karen, a middle-aged woman from Belize, who was recommended by a friend. Overnight, it became apparent to me that I could no longer leave Geoff while I raced out to buy groceries. Having Karen work four hours a day meant assistance bathing and dressing him.

Geoff wasn't happy about the arrangement at first, but Karen was so quiet and patient that he quickly got used to her. She was also strong and skilled, so he trusted her to help him. But he really warmed to her when she gently massaged his shoulders and feet, calming him when he became anxious. He liked to have her sit somewhere behind him, out of sight but always available when he needed her.

We hadn't been out since returning from New York, although a few friends had stopped by to visit. But after a week of chill and rain, we woke up to a sunny Sunday morning and I decided to take Geoff out for lunch. For the first time in nearly a week, he rode down the chair lift. I'd already carefully prepared the route: I'd set up the transport chair at the foot of the stairs, opened the kitchen door, unlocked the garden gate, raised the garage door and parked the car in the driveway, leaving the passenger door open. The transfer from the wheelchair to the car went smoothly and we headed off to Geoff's favorite Mexican restaurant, El Cholo.

The valet parker assisted me with the wheelchair, and a waiter got us situated at a corner table. We had a marvelous lunch, complete with a margarita for Geoff. With our heads together, laughing and talking, it felt like we were on a date.

But that night, I awakened around two o'clock, this time my face wet with tears from a vivid dream in which I was lost in a woods. My leg brushed against Geoff's and I was struck with a piercing fear that one night I would no longer have his leg to brush against. I smoothed my hand along his back, feeling his warmth. A fresh flood of silent tears burned my cheeks. Geoff was sound asleep for once, and I was the one frightened and anxious. I lay with my hand on his shoulder, craving the comfort Geoff needed whenever he asked me to keep my hand on him so he could sleep.

One night, when I'd almost fallen asleep, Geoff woke me up to ask when Harry would be arriving to take us to the airport. "Where do you think we're going?" I asked.

"Moscow for the wedding."

"We're not going to Moscow for a wedding. We don't even know anyone in Moscow." For the next hour or so I fielded questions about the nonexistent trip.

"I hope the flight is nonstop," he said. "Do you think we have to refuel in Minneapolis?"

"Maybe," I said finally. "Let's get some sleep until Harry gets here."

The following morning, Geoff was still convinced we were going to Moscow and had missed our flight. "There aren't that many direct flights each day," he said, his whispery voice full of reproach. Not until Karen was feeding him lunch did he acknowledge that he might have been dreaming.

There were so many signs of decline, all of them

coming on fast. His voice was often so faint I could barely hear him. Sometimes only his lips moved, struggling to form words with no sound. I urged him to tell me anything he really wanted me to know while he could still communicate. Would he like to make changes in how he managed his investments while he could still instruct someone? He shook his head. "Don't make me talk," he whispered.

On October 13, I managed to combine visits with Dr. Portera and Dr. Bordelon for the same day so that I wouldn't have to get Geoff to UCLA twice in one week. He had to fast prior to our morning appointment, so I packed up a container of yogurt, his Phase II powder and regular meds. I remained calm, knowing that any show of anxiousness on my part doomed us, but he was listless and not at all responsive when I tried to talk with him.

In the examining room at UCLA, it was difficult getting his EKG, blood pressure and other tests completed. Fortunately there were no cognitive tests scheduled, because Geoff would not have been able to respond. We spent twenty minutes in a bathroom trying to get a urine sample. He became frustrated with himself and me. "I can't do anything on demand!" His whisper was vehement and heartbreaking. Everything was a struggle.

While the research assistant was drawing blood samples, I took the opportunity to privately discuss the Phase II medication with Dr. Bordelon. I'd come armed with newly published reports on another medication tested on PSP patients, wondering if Geoff should switch programs. It was clear that he had declined in the three months he'd been in the Phase II testing program. Possibly he was taking only a placebo, or the "miracle potion" was simply ineffective in slowing the relentless progression of the disease.

The alternate testing program that was touting such great results was only twelve weeks long, with just twelve patients enrolled, and they had symptoms of various conditions, not just PSP. Nonetheless, Dr. Bordelon agreed that it was worth looking into and said she would speak to Dr. Portera about it. She also asked if I needed home assistance and offered to make some suggestions. I realized I probably looked as harried and troubled as I felt. I managed to hold back tears, but it was hard seeing the concern in her eyes. She was young enough to be my daughter. As strong and capable as I knew she was, I somehow didn't want to worry her.

Dr. Portera examined Geoff and it was obvious he was surprised by the considerable decline since the last visit. Geoff admitted that he got anxious and sometimes cried out when he couldn't see me, and that he sometimes forgot that I was just in the next room. I let Geoff do all the talking, most of it in a whisper, and nodded when Dr. Portera looked to me for confirmation.

It occurred to me that on our previous visit to Dr. Portera, Geoff and I had walked into the examining room arm in arm, joking and laughing. My heart broke seeing Geoff slumped in the wheelchair, looking confused, unable to perform such simple tasks as clapping his hands together.

October 26—I talk with Mari and Nancy and learn that Ed and Josh have both declined in the past few weeks, too. Mari has full-time help but, like me, Nancy is trying to manage on her own because Josh refuses to have home help. Unfortunately, Nancy is now also having cancer treatment. Josh, like Geoff, is having considerable difficulty walking or speaking.

Josh's brother, a doctor, has suggested to Nancy that she look into hospice home care, which is funded by Medicare. "Hospice now?" is barely out of my mouth before Nancy says, "Wait, let me explain. Josh is eligible because his disease is terminal, with no treatment or medication available, and he would receive only palliative care. He's also unable to feed, clothe, bathe, walk or use a toilet without assistance. He requires full-time care. His brother called a hospice service and we have an appointment with a social worker and admissions nurse."

Nancy gave me all the information about the particular company her brother-in-law recommended. I called them to make an appointment. Once I made the initial call, everything happened very quickly. Even though it was a weekend, a social worker made an appointment to assess Geoff.

The following day, an admissions nurse and a registered nurse arrived for a three-hour visit. The RN checked Geoff's vital signs, made a list of his medications and filled out a lengthy medical history. The admissions nurse spoke with Dr. Portera and spent considerable time creating a treatment chart. Dr. Bordelon had already assured me that signing on for hospice care would not negate Geoff's participation in the Phase II drug program. In terms of care and medication, there would be no change in his treatment program.

Geoff clearly fit all the requirements for hospice care, yet it seemed to me too early to sign on for it. I asked a lot of questions and still felt unsure about my decision. I insisted we didn't need morphine, oxygen tanks and various other types of equipment and supplies, but was told some of it was mandatory. "We'll want it here on hand in case of emergency."

Hospice arrived just before Thanksgiving, bringing

with it floods of paperwork, rotating staff, medication and equipment. I agreed to the minimum service: a visit by a nurse once a week, and a health aide twice a week to assist with bathing. I stored the oxygen machine and other "just in case" equipment in the guest room closet, out of sight until we "might" need it. Medication with boldface warning labels scared me. I stashed a small box containing morphine behind lettuce and carrots in the vegetable crisper. I didn't want to see it.

The following day, we had the first scheduled visit from the RN. We also had a visit from Gwen, the health aide who would assist with bathing. It turned out she and Karen knew each other through previous hospice clients. Together, they got Geoff seated on the bench in the shower. What a relief not to have to worry about having him fall!

The hospice doctor, with impeccable manners and an ability to ask sensitive questions without alarming Geoff, spent about a half hour with us. When I walked the doctor to the door, I told him I wasn't certain I'd made a good decision in seeking hospice home care so soon. While Geoff had declined in the last few weeks, death was clearly far from imminent. The doctor surprised me by saying that wasn't necessarily true, that any number of situations could arise, including pneumonia. It was up to me to know in advance what Geoff would want and have a signed document on hand. I could feel my ears close down as he spoke, but I kept nodding that I understood.

After both he and Karen left, I went to the mailbox and discovered circulars from Forest Lawn, Advanced Care Networks and the Neptune Society. Clearly our enrollment in hospice wasn't a secret.

I went upstairs to check on Geoff, who was sitting on the couch, the television turned low. He was pale, his eyes staring. I reached for his hands, which were icy cold, and fitted them inside his sheepskin-lined suede mittens. He could barely speak but said he was tired. I tried to walk him to the bedroom but couldn't. I transferred him to the chair for the short trip to the bed. He curled up and I covered him. He looked so shrunken, his skin gray. I was certain he was reacting to the doctor's visit and all the home care activity. He had to know what was happening.

"They're just here to give us a hand. It's safer. You'll be more comfortable." He gave no response. I sat on the edge of the bed, stroking his shoulder until he drifted off to sleep.

I made myself a cup of tea and took a walk in the garden, sucking in deep breaths and shedding tears. I could only hope I'd done the right thing in ordering hospice care. How could all this have happened only a month after our trip to New York and Nashville? Yet, once I understand the nature of hospice care, I recognized that it was an appropriate choice for our situation. For his comfort and safety, Geoff required the level of home care hospice would provide.

Each incremental change had come in its own time. When the need presented itself, we dealt with it. The walker. Grab bars. The stair lift. Transport chair. Wheelchair. Home help. Hospice. When something became necessary, we got it—and quickly got used to it. We tried not to think about a time when we didn't need the assistance, the apparatus, or whatever else had become impossible to do without. Instead, I was grateful aid was available and that we had access to it.

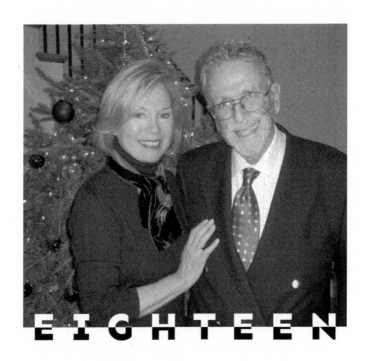

EIGHTEEN

"A ROOM WITH A VIEW"

An editor at the London *Sunday Telegraph*, who was familiar with my book *The Bunny Years*, the twenty-five-year history of Playboy clubs, tracked me down to write a piece on the new Playboy Club casino opening in London on Old Park Lane near the site of the original 1960s-era club. I accepted the assignment but had to work quickly to meet the deadline. I propped my laptop on my knees and sat on the couch next to Geoff to write while he watched CNBC.

I took a break to feed him a quick dinner and then went back to work. After tucking him in for the night, I sat on the edge of the bed and read the draft aloud. He made a few whispered comments, and I spent another hour or so polishing. I was feeling very pleased with myself when I emailed the piece at midnight, meeting my deadline.

Payment for the article was wired directly into my bank account, and I wasted no time in spending it on a zero-gravity recliner for Geoff. Sitting on a couch encased in pillows to prevent him from sliding to the floor and using a bathroom stool as a footrest hadn't been very comfortable for him. I positioned the recliner in a corner of the bedroom facing the television, where I could see him from my desk in the den, a perfect arrangement. The master bedroom was sunny and bright, with French doors and casement windows looking out on the pool and garden. It occurred to me that Geoff's wife, Barbara, had spent many years lying on a daybed next to those very windows, looking out at the same view. The recliner made such a huge difference in Geoff's level of comfort that his general health seemed to improve. It was also far easier to transfer him into the wheelchair.

I began feeling less secure about my hospice decision. Nancy confided that Josh had declined hospice home care, instead agreeing to nursing assistance eight hours a day. Should that have been our choice? My doubts increased. I worried that I'd been too hasty and considered canceling hospice care in favor of hiring more home help. But then, I couldn't really base my decision on a comparison with Ed and Josh, because they each had a different prognosis than Geoff. Even though they both appeared to be more physically disabled when we first met, Geoff's decline was more precipitous. I continued with hospice, but kept in mind that I could cancel it at any time.

One Friday afternoon, after a full week of rotating hospice staff in the house, Geoff and I were on our own, relishing some quiet time alone together. Karen had left for the day and wouldn't return until the following morning. I read to Geoff until he became drowsy and said he wanted to nap. Rather than shift him to the bed, I reclined his chair almost flat and covered him with a blanket before going to my desk in the next room.

Perhaps fifteen minutes later, I heard an odd whirring sound in the bedroom and hurried to check on him. To my horror, I saw Geoff sprawled on the floor, his hand clutching the remote control with his thumb clamped on the lift button. The recliner was almost erect and still rising, making the gentle whirring sound I'd heard. I pried the remote from Geoff's hand and stopped the chair, which by then was fully perpendicular to the floor.

I kneeled beside Geoff, who was lying facedown, trembling. He looked up at me and grinned. "Took a ride. Couldn't stop."

"I can see that." I had to smile. "Are you okay? Did you hit your head?"

"Just slid. No somersault."

I helped him roll onto his side, thankful I'd removed his eyeglasses before he napped. There was a small rug burn on his cheek, but he looked otherwise undamaged. "Sorry, Geoff, it was my fault. I shouldn't have left the remote where you could reach it. How do you feel?"

"Stay with me," he whispered.

He was still smiling, but his eyes were anxious. I slid a pillow under our heads and covered us with the blanket. We'd both had a scare and needed time to calm down. The erect chair looming above us was a funny sight that made us laugh, but it was also a frightening reminder that Geoff could have been seriously hurt. We lay on the floor together, talking quietly as the sun faded into evening. He assured me he was feeling no pain, that his shoulder was fine. Daphne joined us, curling up on my chest, purring contentedly.

Eventually Geoff said he wanted to sit up and watch the news. "Isn't it time for supper?"

I turned on the television and left Geoff lying on the floor while I telephoned our neighbor. Stuart arrived within a minute.

"No more gymnastics, okay, pal?" Stuart said as he helped me get Geoff back in the recliner.

"Where's the fun in that?" Geoff asked. I made sure the incident wouldn't happen again by carefully tucking the remote control into a pocket behind the chair.

October 30, 2010—We've been invited for dinner at the Hedisons', a long-planned get-together with Kimberley and David Brody, visiting from San Francisco, Corky and Mike Stoller, Seymore Englander, and Bridget and David's daughter, Serena, who is in LA working on a documentary project. These are among our favorite friends, and Geoff insists he's feeling well enough to go. We begin getting ready at 4:00 p.m. for the 7:30 dinner. Before Karen leaves for the day, we manage to get Geoff in the shower, trim his beard, clip his nails, brush his teeth and then bathe and shampoo him. The entire process takes well over an hour, and he's exhausted by the time we finish. I wrap him in a robe and have him take a nap in the recliner while I bathe. I struggle on my own to dress him in black cord pants and a black turtleneck. He looks great. I sense that he's feeling agitated and ask him if he wants to take his "calming pill" early. "Please," he says.

Stuart helps me get Geoff into the stair lift, then the transport chair at the foot of the stairs and out to the car. It takes us twenty minutes before he's safely strapped in, ready to go. I lock up and leave lights on in the house and garden in case I'm on my own when we come home in the dark. We're on the road by 7:25 for the five-minute drive to the Hedisons' house. I manage to get the transport chair out of the trunk, but Serena helps me get Geoff into the house. It's exciting to see everyone, and Geoff glows with pleasure. I position the wheelchair so he's at the center of the party. He can't speak, but at least he can hear everything. The food is great, and I even give Geoff a few sips of red wine.

Geoff tries hard to enter into the conversation, and I manage to repeat some of what he whispers to me. Mike is leaving for NY in the morning to cast his new Broadway musical, and Geoff would love to talk with him about it. At one point, Mike can't think of the first name of a musician, and Geoff triumphantly supplies the name, "Irving." Everyone laughs and Geoff is very pleased with himself.

We're on our own coming home. The neighbors are at a Halloween party. Somehow, having consumed a glass or two of good red myself, I manage to get Geoff into the transport chair, inside the house, into the chair lift, then haul the transport chair upstairs and get him back into it. I race down to park the car in the garage and lock up before putting Geoff to bed. It's a struggle but all worth it!

Geoff was so thrilled with his new zero-gravity

recliner that we built our social life around it. I rearranged the furniture and even set up a round table with two bistro chairs near the French doors. The bedroom became our breakfast room, dining room, living room and media center—and where we began doing all of our entertaining. We instituted our own happy hour, where friends could drop in for coffee or drinks at the end of the day and enjoy our company without seeing medications and handicap equipment. Laughter. Music. It was a time for stories and fond memories. Friends arrived from San Francisco. London. Minneapolis. New York. Santa Barbara. Wine and Sam Adams pilsner were on tap, along with cakes and cookies. Martinis, of course.

Dr. Bordelon had suggested that Geoff might benefit from a voice amplifier. I found a portable device online that came with a headset. The headband was comfortable to wear, and he liked pulling the sponge-covered mic within an inch of his mouth—he dubbed it "the Madonna." He delighted in showing off for guests, putting on a radio announcer's voice and doing sound effects. His voice grew so strong, I had to turn down the volume. It was great being able to have sporadic conversations with him again and hearing the wonderful sound of his voice.

Geoff looked forward to our happy hour, his eagerness apparent as he did playful sound checks on his "Madonna" before friends arrived. I concealed medical equipment and medication, lit candles and played soft music, "setting the scene" as Geoff would want it. Among the guests Geoff most enjoyed seeing were London friends Tom and Jeannie Allen, who were staying in Pasadena during Tom's engagement with the Los Angeles Opera.

After they left, I emailed: *Thanks so much for the beautiful orchid! I know it's disconcerting to see Geoff as he is now, but he loved having you visit. He doesn't miss a thing and enjoyed all the stories. You're both such dear friends . . . it's not just anybody we invite to the boudoir for cake and champagne! You really brightened our day and we thank you so much for making the trip into the hills. So good to see you!*

Glenys Roberts, an English journalist who had written for *Los Angeles* magazine in its early years, arrived from London in the company of an Irish priest with a wicked sense of humor. The two brought on tears of laughter with their funny stories. Susan Sullivan and Connell Cowen dropped by, bringing deli sandwiches and wonderful imported beer. Suzanne Childs, an attorney newly retired from the district attorney's office, dropped in often, bringing fruit tarts and Chinese chicken salad. Kay, Kimberley and David, Gil and Miranda, and other old friends and colleagues stopped in for coffee and drinks, enlivening our afternoons with cheerful conversation. I encouraged these visits and asked everyone to spread the word among our friends that Geoff thrived on seeing people.

Those visits were good for me, too. I was becoming more isolated, just as Geoff was, and craved that social outlet. Laughter was a tonic, easing tension. Good conversation among friends nourished the mind and soul, lifting the gloom I too often felt sitting alone with Geoff, holding his hand while he watched television. When we were by ourselves, it was only when I was reading aloud to him that I felt we were fully engaged with each other. Talking, even with the amplifier, was still hard work for him and he could only manage it for a short time each day.

Everyone told me what all caregivers hear: Take care of yourself. Yet I considered myself agile and strong and felt more capable than I probably was. I took chances I shouldn't have. Several times a night, I would load Geoff into the transport chair to take him the short distance to the bathroom. It was arduous and too often I took shortcuts, urging him to walk the few steps to the toilet.

If he abruptly stopped moving, we'd both get rattled. He'd stiffen, freeze in place and begin sagging in my arms. Worse, by the time I eventually got him to the bathroom, he was too traumatized to use the toilet. Other times, Geoff would become difficult and demanding, insisting that he could walk—and would occasionally try to get up and walk on his own. Several times, he slid onto the floor and I would struggle for an hour to get him back in the bed. On one occasion, I gave up and lay down on the floor next to him. Sharing a pillow and blanket, we slept until dawn.

I knew I was straining myself and that the tension was getting to me. I had terrible stomach pains and aching joints and muscles. I was losing weight. Sometimes I felt dizzy. I increased Karen's work schedule from four to six hours a day. Having her on duty meant I didn't have to jump up whenever Geoff was thirsty, wanted chocolate, a blanket or pillow, needed the channel changed, his mittens put back on, had to be reseated or taken to the bathroom. I also forced myself to play by the rules, using the gait belt to transfer Geoff to the transport chair instead of trying to walk him.

Lisa Seidman, a screenwriter friend, proposed we partner on writing a script based on one of my novels. We kept to a regular schedule, working at my desk, where I could keep an eye on Geoff. I checked on him periodically and he seemed content, knowing he could get my attention if he needed it. In fact, having Lisa's company while working on the screenplay had an unexpected benefit: my aches and pains, probably caused by physical and mental strain, eased considerably.

But even during the hours Karen worked at the house, I couldn't really leave Geoff alone. If I was gone too often, or too long, I paid for it when I got home. Geoff would turn his head away and whisper that I no longer loved him and wanted to be out of the house as much as possible. Or he would become so agitated and delay me with so many excuses and demands that I ended up not going out. Oddly enough, I remembered Geoff telling me years earlier that Barbara had behaved in that same manner.

"She couldn't help it," Geoff had said. "I was her lifeline. It was a neediness she couldn't control, any more than her MS." I reminded myself of his comments about Barbara every time I had to negotiate with him about going out somewhere.

If I was Geoff's lifeline, Candy became mine. Even though Geoff liked Karen very much, he was most comfortable with Candy. With her on hand, he didn't resent my absence as much. Therefore, I used Wednesdays to buy groceries, fill the gas tank, go to the bank and post office and do any other errands or appointments I could fit in.

Otherwise, I spent most of my days attending to Geoff and working at my desk whenever he was napping. In the late afternoon, when we didn't have happy hour guests, I read to him before dinner, then we'd watch a film and I'd put him to bed around 8:30 p.m.

That was our day, that was our life, and the tedium was more onerous for him than me. Sitting all day, even in his glorious recliner, didn't provide him with the stimulation he craved.

Geoff insisted on going to New York for the Christmas holidays. Well, why not? I discussed it with Dr. Bordelon and Dr. Portera, who both indicated it would be fine to take our Phase II medications with us as long as we returned in time for our next scheduled appointment. I spoke with the hospice team and was told, "If that's what you want to do, it's up to you."

I booked our flight using miles and upgrades, and did it despite suspecting everyone was secretly thinking, "That woman is stark, raving *nuts!*"

But I was also counting on my personal army of supporters. Harry would take us to the airport and stay in our house while we were gone. My brother Orlyn, nephew Tom and his wife would be in New York when we arrived. Tim and David booked tickets to New York to give me a hand over the New Year's holiday. The staff at the apartment building could be counted on for occasional assistance. I also hired home help through an agency that came highly recommended. Honestly, what could go wrong?

December 16—Our flight to NY was smooth and easy ... what a relief! American Airlines makes everything comfortable. We're first on, last off. I packed lots of treats. Whenever Geoff got restive, I gave him a cookie or some peanut brittle. An airline porter wheeled Geoff to the baggage area, then out to the limo pickup without mishap.

When we arrived at our apartment, Orlyn, who'd flown in from Minneapolis that afternoon for business meetings, and Tom and Barb were on hand to greet us. They'd decorated a tree, bought flowers and had a bottle of wine open . . . I literally wept with joy. We then all went out for dinner in the neighborhood with Geoff in the sturdy new wheelchair that I bought online and had shipped to the apartment. Orlyn and Tom had it assembled and ready to use. Friday, my nephew wheeled Geoff to Rockefeller Plaza while Barb and I shopped for fun gifts for young grandnieces and grandnephews. Then we all met at Birdland. What a treat this has been to have "family" help for a few days. I had enough time to rush here and there to the market, drugstore, etc. to lay in supplies for the duration.

The real test began once I was on my own. The home care I had lined up went AWOL. I left numerous messages but got no response from the woman I'd hired by telephone. The agency said they had no one else available short-term over the holidays. I decided not to waste more time trying to find someone. Besides, I felt uncomfortable leaving Geoff's care to someone I didn't have time to vet, who might do him more harm than good.

I had two business meetings scheduled that I put off because I couldn't rely on busy doormen to look in on him regularly. It wasn't a surprise that Geoff required more assistance than he did when we were in New York in September, but he was even more debilitated than he'd been only days earlier in Los Angeles. I would have canceled the trip if I'd more accurately assessed his condition before we left.

In Los Angeles, I had Candy, Harry and Stuart only a telephone call away, Karen to help six hours a day, an agency that could always supply additional assistance on short notice and hospice care already set up. I also had the luxury of space and the ideal setup with the bed, recliner and bathroom in close proximity. I had none of that available to me in New York. Geoff was too weak to speak or walk, and could only sit up if propped with pillows.

The biggest problem turned out to be Geoff's hallucinations during the night. I would awaken to find him thrashing his legs and whispering nonsensically.

"We're going to miss the plane! Call Harry to pick us up."

"Get me up, get me up, justice must be done."

"When do we get to Moscow?"

"The wedding, we'll miss the wedding."

"Did you count the books? Did they take the cartoons?"

I'd cup his face in my hands and look into his eyes, trying to get through to him. There was no wedding, no trip to Moscow, no books to be counted and Harry wouldn't be picking us up because we were in New York. Sometimes he was so insistent about getting up that he managed to swing his legs off the bed. By the time I'd shoved him back on the bed, arranged his arms, legs and head comfortably, I was shaking with exertion and frustration.

"Geoff, please understand that if we carry on like this tonight I won't be able to take care of you during the day."

"I had to take care of Barbara five or six times a night."

"I know, but you were thirty years younger and she was ninety pounds lighter!"

"I'll soon be gone. Then I won't bother you."

"Please don't say things like that. I want you with me no matter what!"

One night I awakened close to midnight, hearing Geoff whisper, "Help me, help, help." I leapt to my feet and saw that he was about to fall out of bed. He was hallucinating, insisting it was time to get up. I turned on the light, showed him the clock and swung his legs back in bed. He insisted I was lying, that we had to "get up or we're going to be late getting home."

I opened the window blinds. "Please, stop this craziness! It's dark outside. It's midnight!"

And so it went, night after night. He couldn't turn over or adjust his body, so he wasn't able to sleep and became even more disoriented. Angry, exhausted and unable to go back to sleep myself, I sat up in bed, reminding myself not to take out my frustration on Geoff. We often remained awake most of the night, dozing off as dawn filtered through the window blinds.

I realized that the trip had been a huge miscalculation on my part. *What was I thinking?* We needed to go back to Los Angeles—but how to get him there? I was terrified of a flight home with Geoff agitated and hallucinating. I even considered renting a car, buckling him in and just barreling across country, ice storms and blizzards be damned. I'd made a terrible mistake and didn't know what to do.

Miraculously, Geoff had a turnabout. After five unbearable nights, the fog of agitation and confusion lifted and he woke up smiling and coherent. We celebrated with lunch at a nearby restaurant and made plans for Christmas Eve. I rang Krista, one of my closest friends in New York, who was recovering from another round of chemo treatment, and asked her to join us in carol singing at the Irving Berlin house on Beekman Place. Afterward, we walked back to our apartment for champagne and a light supper. We made it an early evening, none of us wanting to push the boundaries of well-being.

The biggest boost for us was the arrival of Tim and David, who were able to stay for a week in a friend's nearby vacant apartment. Geoff smiled the moment they walked in. Both are tall, strong and able, and Geoff felt very secure in their company. Tim's medical background helped us through a couple of mishaps, and I knew Geoff would be safe in their care while I went out.

I took full advantage of their afternoon visits, cramming in the postponed business meetings and enjoying the city. What a pleasure to walk fast, jump on a bus, take a subway, shop and meet friends without worrying about the clock. I met Cynthia, my literary agent, for tea, then stayed on for a glass of wine, talking nonstop, grateful that I didn't have to rush home. When I returned, Geoff was tucked into the Eames chair, wrapped in a blanket with a pillow behind his head, watching a film with Tim and David.

On New Year's Eve, David, who is a chef, prepared a banquet for the four of us: filet mignon and grilled vegetables. Afterward, we watched an Academy screener of *The King's Speech* before welcoming in the New Year. Tim and David helped me put Geoff to bed before they left. When I was certain Geoff was asleep and safely barricaded with pillows, I took a short walk. At the end of our street I looked across the East River, where the Pepsi-Cola sign glowed red like a giant Christmas bauble against a starlit sky. The fireworks were finished, a new year begun.

My eyes watered, not with tears but with the chill of the night. I was glad that, despite the difficulties and challenges of those first few days, we had made the trip. Who knew if Geoff would be back in New York next Christmas?

My lips moved in prayerful words that sounded like a promise I was making to myself. *Patience. Kindness . . . Treasure the joy of precious moments together . . . Be gentle. No harsh words you'll regret, because you can't take them back, not ever.*

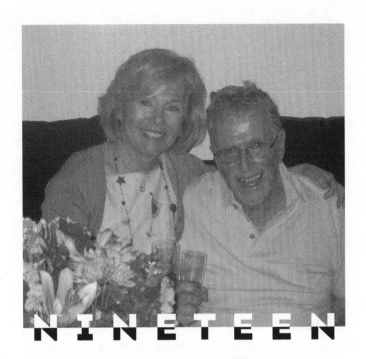

NINETEEN

"THE VERY THOUGHT OF YOU"

January 12, 2011—*Within a week of our return from New York, we have another appointment with Dr. Bordelon at UCLA. The session is cut short because Geoff is weak, unable to speak, and therefore the physical and cognitive tests can't be completed. While Geoff is in an examining room struggling through an EKG, I speak privately with Dr. Bordelon. To my surprise, and probably hers, I burst into tears. "It's a bad day," I sob. "Everything is moving so quickly."*

I'd managed to hold back emotion during our doctor's appointments, but at that moment, I knew we had reached the end. It was pointless to continue the Phase II testing program. Despite warnings not to do so, we'd pinned such hopes on it. Every morning when I opened that packet of "miracle potion" and dissolved the powder into water, I secretly expected it to be the magic dose that led to a cure.

I wished for that cure every day and prayed for it at night. For me, those packets contained the Salk vaccine, penicillin and chicken soup of my dreams, and I couldn't let it go. I sobbed for myself and then I sobbed some more because I would have to tell Geoff we were bowing out of the clinical trial.

The decision to discontinue the program was also another reminder of how much Geoff had declined in six months. That morning, he had been less responsive than usual when I gave him a sponge bath, brushed his teeth and dressed him. I opened the kitchen and garden doors, pulled the car out and called Stuart to help me get Geoff down the stairs, into the wheelchair and out to the car, still hoping. But everything had been more difficult. After our appointment with Dr. Bordelon, I was terribly depressed as I loaded Geoff back into the car. He, on the other hand, looked upbeat, perhaps because the ordeal of the morning was over. I decided to wait before mentioning to him that we were discontinuing the Phase II drug trial.

On our way home, I stopped to pick up mail from my post office box. As I had in the past, I left Geoff in the car listening to music, telling him I'd be right back. I kept an eye on our parked car, visible through the large plate-glass windows, as I sprinted in and out of the post office in under a minute. But just as I reached the car, I saw that Geoff was opening the passenger door.

"We need groceries," he said, his voice surprisingly strong. "I wanted to help."

"I know, but there isn't a grocery store here."

He looked befuddled. "I thought you were in a grocery store."

The following day, all signs of confusion and weakness vanished. If only he'd been so alert and engaged at UCLA! His appetite was robust, and once again I was able to walk him from the bed to the recliner. His voice was vibrant, even without using the amplifier. I began reading chapters of *Three Chords for Beauty's Sake*, Tom Nolan's book on Artie Shaw, to him. Geoff would frequently interject a story about one of the musicians or talk about Artie. I wondered if he was actually benefiting from discontinuing the Phase II drug.

While it lasted, I took advantage of his ability to speak again. He liked my suggestion that he donate his collection of *Los Angeles* magazines to the UCLA library. It seemed fitting since he had developed a prototype for the magazine while earning his master's degree at UCLA in 1960.

I asked him if he had kept any original documents or handwritten papers about the magazine's startup that he could also donate. He thought there might be some folders in the file cabinets in his office. I offered to help him go through the drawers, but he said they were locked and he'd forgotten where the key was. "Don't bother looking for it," he said. "You'll never find it."

Geoff continued to rebound. He seemed energized

and purposeful, taking renewed interest in his stock portfolio. Several times, he asked me to retrieve books or papers from his office and became impatient if I couldn't quickly find things for him. He seemed in a hurry.

On Wednesday, after Karen left, I asked Candy to keep an eye on Geoff while I attended my book club meeting. Before I left, I made lunch for both of them and reminded Geoff not to ask Candy to help him stand or move around. I told him I wouldn't be gone long and would read to him when I returned.

My birthday was coming up in two days and my book club friends surprised me with cards, gifts and a cake. Raleigh, who had served a delicious chicken salad, packed up fruit and cake for me to take home. When I arrived back, Candy was in the kitchen ironing. The moment she saw me, she started crying.

"What's wrong? Is Geoff all right?" I asked, alarmed.

"I help him go to his office," she said tearfully. "He wanted to find a key."

"Did he find it?"

"Oh, yes. He wanted to throw away things. Please don't be mad at him. It's not right for me to say no to Mr. Miller. I bring him bags and hold for him."

On my way upstairs I saw bulging black plastic bags and cartons stuffed with files on the landing. Geoff was settled in his recliner watching CNBC. I showed him my gifts and told him I'd brought home birthday cake and fruit salad. "Candy said she helped you in your office. Is everything okay?"

"Fine. I threw away some stuff."

"You must've found the key."

"I remembered where I put it."

"You should've waited for me. I would've helped you."

"I wanted to spare you. Don't bother looking in the bags. Candy will take them out."

Our casual banter was surreal given that Geoff hadn't been able to converse this easily in well over a year. He was fully engaged, his eyes alert. He was speaking in a normal voice. He'd crossed his legs and was sitting erect, his posture suggesting he was in full control. I realized that in order to accomplish so much in the short time I was gone, he'd asked for Candy's help the moment I left. He'd planned this job for when he knew he'd be alone with her in the house. Why?

"What was so urgent? Now Candy's upset. You could've waited."

"Leave it. It's my business."

"But I'm concerned about what you've thrown away. Personal letters and private papers, fine—but what else are you throwing out? I'm going to have to take a look."

"Don't!"

"You can watch me. We'll go through it together. I promise I won't read or look at anything you don't want me to see."

I waited until Candy left for the day before I began opening the bags and cartons. I had misgivings about disregarding his wishes until I started coming across essential documents, certificates and records, including our marriage license and the original deed to the house. He'd clearly dumped the contents of entire file drawers into the bags Candy held open. Where had he gotten the strength?

"Why did you throw this? We need this!" I grew more upset the more I found.

I tipped one bag on its side and a small red-and-gold Cartier box fell out, spilling a shiny link bracelet onto the floor. I stared at it, then at the card wedged inside the box: K—*With all my love*, G. I'd never seen the bracelet but knew it had to be the anniversary gift Geoff bought a few years earlier, then misplaced before he could give it to me. The gift box had been propped open inside an empty bank check carton, hidden away in a desk drawer until that moment.

"You didn't even look at what you were throwing away!" I shouted angrily. "What were you thinking?"

He looked surprised by what I'd found, but was still defiant. He glared at me, half rising to his feet, shouting, "I can do what I want! Throw everything! Get rid of it! It's mine! I don't need it, don't want it!"

I was stunned by his vehemence. "Sorry, I know there's personal stuff here, but some of this can't be thrown. I need it."

I set aside the files that were important to keep, but refilled the bags with clippings, magazines, keepsakes, old letters and other personal materials that he had every right to discard, including bundles of letters, address books and photographs that belonged to Barbara. I snatched a few items of hers that I knew her son and daughter would treasure, but discarded the rest.

Geoff appeared mollified, yet a cloud hung over both of us that didn't dissipate, even after we ate birthday cake and I read to him. I made light of finding the bracelet, thanking him for the timely birthday gift, and was rewarded with a grudging smile. But I felt his resentment, and the warmth and intimacy we usually shared was absent. He was subdued when I put him to bed that night, his energy spent. For the first time in weeks, he slept through the night.

The following morning, I awakened to hear Geoff whispering. I leaned close as he murmured softly, "What's holding us up from leaving?"

"We're not going anywhere. Where do you want to go?"

"Home."

"We're home. Look out the window. That's our garden." I kissed him, then put my hand to his forehead. He felt feverish, his skin clammy. "Are you all right?"

"I want to go home." He clamped his eyes shut and I saw tears on his cheek. I also heard a wheezing sound in his chest. I quickly telephoned the hospice nurse.

Karen arrived while I was on the phone and helped me get him to the bathroom. "He's very sick. I think he might have pneumonia," she said. The nurse confirmed it when she arrived. She called the hospice doctor, then asked for some of the medications stored in the refrigerator.

"But it can't be that serious! He was in such great shape yesterday, even cleaning his office."

She nodded. "It goes that way, sometimes. A burst of energy before the end."

"The end! No! It's not the end! We need to get him to the hospital!"

"If you want to make that call, you need to do it quickly. It's up to you to terminate hospice care."

Then I understood. Within minutes of my call, paramedics arrived to take Geoff to the hospital. I grabbed my emergency folder and jumped into the car, calling Harry, Tim and David as I drove.

When I arrived inside the emergency entrance, a doctor was waiting for me. "Mrs. Miller? It's urgent. You know you've got a DNR in place?"

"No, I canceled it!"

"With hospice, but not here. Follow me!"

I stood next to the gurney, holding Geoff's hand, sobbing a plea not to leave me. "Please, please, not now, not after yesterday! We need more time! You can't go like this, not now!"

His face was ashen, his body hooked up to an array of machines and monitors. I was beside myself with fear. How could this have come on so quickly?

Harry arrived, then Tim and David. We stood together for hours until Geoff slowly began to respond. He was moved to a hospital room and I sat alone at his bedside, holding his hand, whispering to him. "Stay with me, please stay with me. I can't let you go like this."

Throughout the night, sitting in the pale glow of the flickering monitors, comforted by heartbeat sounds of steady beeping, I had hours to reflect on what had transpired the day before. I realized he'd been on a mission, summoning the last of his strength and energy to "tidy up" before going on his way, just as my mother had. He'd quite plainly let me know it was time for him to go "home." I felt his rebuke that I'd interrupted his journey.

I was ashamed I'd behaved so blindly and stupidly. Why had I forced the issue when I could have handled things so much more gracefully? There'd been no need to lash out, to humiliate him by ripping through those bags. He was letting me know he didn't need *things* anymore. There was no reason for me to show him that I did. All I'd done was point up the great divide growing between us; he was leaving, while I was staying behind. I was determined to make up for my behavior, to give him the love and kindness I'd promised myself I would. There couldn't be any regrets. It had to be a "good" goodbye.

When he finally came around, it was as though the sun had come out after a rainstorm. There was a look of wonder in his eyes, a sense of surprise when he saw me. He was weak, but there was warmth in his smile. He rallied even more when a few close friends stopped by for brief visits.

Miranda Lipton took me for a birthday lunch at a French café near the hospital, but otherwise I stayed close to Geoff. He was calm, accepting of everything the hospital staff did. I fed him malted milks and read to him, sitting with him for long hours. He didn't want to talk and seemed only mildly interested that I was there with him. It was as though he was a casual visitor, just being polite until he could take his leave.

After three days, I took him home and reinstated hospice care. He was disoriented and hallucinating much of the time, with little sense of place or time. I awoke at six a.m. to find him trying to get out of bed.

"Hurry, I have to get dressed," he whispered urgently. "Time to go home."

For long periods he sat staring blankly, barely acknowledging I was with him, reading or holding his hand. Steve Selcer called to say he would drop by for a visit. I had to remind Geoff that Steve was his stepson. Yet, when Steve arrived, Geoff smiled and enjoyed the visit.

"I'm glad he came by," he whispered later. "He needed to talk."

February 5—Geoff was restless all night. I was up five times to adjust his legs, arms or turn him over. He coughed constantly. At 6:30, I awoke up to find Geoff looking at me, his eyes wide and fearful. "When can we go home?" Later, when I was feeding him oatmeal, he was silent, staring into space. I tapped his cheek and looked into his eyes. "Hey, I know you're in there. Are you okay?" He didn't answer, didn't connect with me. I tried again.

"Do you know where we are?"

"Home? How did we get here?"

Later in the morning, David and Kimberley arrived from San Francisco and stopped in for a visit. Geoff was happy to see them and whispered a few words. I showed them photographs from our South American cruise because our friends are taking the same trip in ten days. It was a shock to see photos of Geoff, standing aboard ship, his arm around me, laughing. He was ill then, and needed assistance, but compared to his condition today, he looked robust and healthy. It was a shock to see the photographs, and hard to deal with the sadness.

February 9—I've prepared Geoff the best I can for my last-minute one-day visit to Minneapolis. Aunty Pat is in hospice at North Memorial Hospital. We're so close and I desperately want to see her before she passes. I've thought about the trip, even checked airline schedules, but Geoff is so newly out of hospital himself that I haven't wanted to make the reservations. Now I know if I don't make the trip I won't see her.

I awaken at 4:00 a.m. and leave for the airport at 4:45 to catch Delta's first flight to Minneapolis. Harry spends the night to be on hand in the morning to keep an eye on Geoff until Candy and Karen arrive. My great fear is weather or maintenance delays, as I have only about six hours available in Minneapolis to visit Aunty Pat. I also want to visit my sister, Sandra, who lives in a special needs residence and is celebrating her 65th birthday. I've tucked a box of chocolates into my shoulder bag for her.

I kiss Geoff goodbye and assure him Harry is awake and available if he needs anything. I race out the door and jump in the car. I can't help it . . . I feel liberated tossing my shoulder bag in the passenger seat and not having to worry about a wheelchair and luggage. The flight is on time. I fall asleep before takeoff and don't wake up until we land. I feel euphoric jumping out of my seat and striding off the plane into the airport, then feel a bit guilty I'm enjoying my freedom so much. Walking fast is one of my greatest pleasures. Orlyn's van is parked at the curb and we pull away the moment I close the car door. My brother drives like I do, swift and assured, and I take pleasure in that, too. We talk about Aunty Pat and I listen closely, even as I take in the familiar wintry vistas. It occurs to me I haven't been in Minnesota since I brought Geoff to the Mayo Clinic in March 2008, nearly three years ago.

Orlyn drops me at the curb near the hospital entrance and tells me he has to attend a meeting. "It'll give you some time alone with Aunty Pat before everyone shows up." The halls are familiar and I barely break stride turning toward the elevator that takes me to the fourth-floor palliative care wing. Aunty Pat is in room 433, the same room Mother was in. I barely recognize my aunt. Her face is tawny gray, her mouth open, her eyes half-mast and unseeing. I drop my bag on the couch and bend low over the bed to kiss her forehead.

"Aunty Pat, it's me. Kathryn. I've come to see you." Stroking her face and holding her hand, I tell her I love her, that she was my fairy godmother and brought so much magic into my life. She'd been my glamorous aunt who smoked, played cards, wore White Shoulders perfume, read racy novels and let me play with her drawers full of costume jewelry. She'd worked in a bridal shop when I was in elementary school and gave me shopworn gowns in tulle and satin, and cocktail dresses in jewel-like colors with fancy hats and long gloves. I spent hours playing dress-up with my friends, organizing neighborhood parades, plays and pageants that featured the dozens of fancy dresses and hats.

Aunty blinks, look at me with her smoky blue eyes, crosses her fingers and touches my cheek, then drifts off again.

A nurse hovers at my shoulder. "Let me know when her son arrives. I called him."

"How's she doing?"

"It's her time. She's dying. The signs are there. That's why I called him."

Glenn and his wife, Susan, arrive minutes later. I call Orlyn to tell him he should return, and he calls David and Kari. We spend the day together sitting around Aunty Pat's bed. In the late afternoon, we share pizza and drink wine, something Pat would've loved. After a brief visit with my sister, Orlyn drops me at the airport. I arrive home at midnight to find Karen sitting in a chair in the darkened bedroom. Geoff is asleep. She leaves and I snuggle up next to him, holding him close.

February 10—My day-long absence was hard on Geoff. He's silent, anxious, staring at me as I open my eyes. I hold his hand under the covers and tell him about my trip. We lie together for nearly an hour before I get up. I know before I even try to get him to his feet that he's not as strong as he was the day before I left. I stack pillows behind and around him so he won't topple over when he sits up. I don't even attempt to get him up on my own. I wait for Karen and Gwen.

February 11—Once again I'm awakened before dawn. Geoff nudges me and whispers that the car has arrived to pick us up. I can barely make out his words. I ask him how he feels.

"Bad."

"Why?"

"I'm dying."

"We all are. We just don't know when."

I stroke his cheek and gently remind him that close friends, who were perfectly healthy when Geoff was diagnosed, have since passed away. "Remember in New York when George cut up your chicken and helped you eat? He died just weeks later. You're still here."

Monday, February 14—Valentine's is an odd day to visit a cemetery to arrange burial for Geoff, but the hospice nurse has made the gentle comment: "If you haven't done so already, it's not too soon to make sure everything is in place." I drive to Holy Cross for my appointment—is this the most expensive place in Christendom to be buried? I'm shocked by the price, even with the "pre-need" discount. Do they have sales? Coupons? My humor black, I wonder if Amazon might offer a better deal. I'm shown the plot where Geoff's parents are buried. There's one plot in that old section available, and it's one tier up, one space over from Rosemary and Ed Miller. Seems too providential. Of course I sign up, then cry all the way home.

February 15—What would I do without Karen? Or Gwen? With six hours of help daily, I now wonder how I could ever have managed on my own. How long before I'll need help around the clock?

Karen and Gwen arrived at 9:30. The three of us worked together to get Geoff into the handicap-equipped shower; a struggle, but worth it. They pampered him with lotions, massaged his feet and hands, combed his hair, brushed his teeth and dressed him, all tasks I formerly did on my own and had difficulty relinquishing to others.

While they changed the linens on the bed, he sat in the reclining chair watching CNBC, seemingly oblivious to the activity swirling around him. Even with home help and hospice care, denial was blissfully at work for him, if not for me. I was still in the grip of my Valentine's Day trip to the cemetery.

As I was about to go downstairs with the basket of laundry, Geoff raised his hand to beckon me. There was a playful look in his eye and my heart melted at the sight of his sweet, lopsided smile. I put down the basket and wrapped my arms around him, giving him a kiss. "Malt," he whispered, his warm breath tickling my ear.

I smiled and gave him another kiss. "I thought you were going to tell me you loved me," I teased.

"Malt," he whispered again, laughter shining in his eyes.

Making a malted milk without shedding tears was more than I could manage. Alone in the kitchen, with Karen upstairs attending to Geoff, I turned on the blender and let my noisy sobs fill the room. Back upstairs, my tears dried, I delivered the malt with a smile. I got a smile in return—along with a halting, whispered request to "make a trade." The smile froze on my face.

I didn't want to make a stock trade and he was aware of it. Our eyes locked and I saw his playful look turn defiant. I knew I couldn't challenge him again. The terrifying aftermath when I'd prevented him from throwing away everything in his office was still fresh in my mind. However foolhardy it was to assist in making the trade, I couldn't deny him his request. Despite bouts of delusion and a long-lost ability to read or write, Geoff was still market savvy and determined to manage his portfolio himself. Making trades, with my assistance, was the last thing he was capable of doing and he wasn't going to relinquish it.

Perhaps his faculties were too clouded to still make the best decisions—but how would I know? I recited columns of numbers from *Barron's* to him, the newsprint blinding, the figures mystifying to me, but Geoff insisted on hearing them. I taught myself to do trades online, where I could look at the maze of numbers, try to make sense of everything and remember what Geoff had taught me, but I hated every minute of it. I will never be a Maria Bartiromo, but if only I could have channeled her just twenty minutes a day!

I made the trade and showed Geoff a printout, proof that I'd followed his instructions. But he insisted on calling an 800 number on speakerphone. He wanted to be sure. I sent Karen to the kitchen while I made the call. Raging inside, I slowly punched up the account numbers. Buying. Selling. It didn't matter. It all terrified me.

What if the trade was a gigantic mistake, a monumental delusion on his part that wiped us out? I prayed that one of the eager, bright young things on the other end of an 800 number would say, "Oh, dear, no! Stop! What are you thinking? Terrible mistake!" It never happened, of course—and looking at the accounts online, I saw nothing but green arrows and rising numbers.

Afterward, with Karen back on duty, I went into the garden, kicked a tree and swore. I'd just made a stock trade at the insistence of a man who'd informed me that Princess Diana had dropped by again—he'd served her a Cosmopolitan. Apparently that was her favorite tipple, although I wouldn't know that for a fact. I seemed never to be around when she visited. He also regularly had close encounters with Kate Moss, whose face reminded him of a kitten's. I could've refused to make trades. I could have lied. I could have been honest with him about my fears, but I couldn't imagine taking from him that singular last sense that he was in charge.

I was playing Russian roulette with our assets, but I also trusted that however impaired Geoff was, his financial acumen was intact. It was largely an emotional response and, however well intentioned, just plain foolish. I'm a businesswoman, but I was worn down and not playing to my strengths. I was lucky in the outcome, because afterward it occurred to me that if Geoff had been so eager to dispose of the contents of his office, where did such an urge stop? Figuratively speaking, could he have impulsively tossed our stock portfolio into a big black bag, too? I should have been more prudent. But then, neither did I remind him I'd been home all afternoon—how had I managed to miss Princess Diana's visit yet again?

While Karen was still on duty, I raced to the bank, post office and grocery store, calming myself in the company of strangers, people who told me to have a good day. I wished them the same in return. What were their days like? Perhaps, in some cases, much like mine. But whatever they were dealing with at home, they wouldn't mention it any more than I would.

February 17—*I'm tired, aching, frustrated and consider canceling my lunch with Susan Sullivan—which will make her laugh since she's always the one to postpone! This is meant to be my birthday lunch three weeks late. It's a beautiful day after a week of rain and we've canceled too many times. Besides, I have an appointment with Fr. Gabriel at All Saints, and I don't want to cancel that. I take a shower and feel better. By the time Karen arrives, I'm dressed and looking forward to lunch.*

Susan takes me to the Polo Lounge and we choose a table in an alcove in the far reaches of the garden. We've been friends for forty-eight years, almost to the day. We met on a gloomy Sunday morning in February 1964 in the New York Playboy Club while both of us were waiting to be photographed in our Bunny costumes (hers blue, mine yellow). At the time, Susan was attending Hofstra University and living at home with her family on Long Island. I was a student at the American Academy of Dramatic Arts and living in my own rent-controlled apartment in a charming Stanford White building on Madison Avenue at Thirtieth Street. Occasionally, when Susan was working full weekend shifts at the Club, she would stay with me.

As we settle back, each with a glass of chardonnay, both of us are more subdued than usual. With Susan's worries about her ninety-four-year-old mother living on her own in Florida and my concerns about Geoff's deteriorating health, conversation is quiet, reflective. Susan reveals feelings about her mother and sister she hadn't mentioned to me before, and I find myself articulating the ache I feel with Geoff pulling away.

Susan gives me a beautiful pin, a duplicate of one she's wearing, and chocolates to bring home to Geoff. It's a long lunch that leaves me feeling calm and settled.

After lunch, I arrived at All Saints with time to spare for a prayer in the chapel before meeting with Fr. Gabri. I went into his office, small and cozily cluttered with books and artwork, and immediately regretted having made the appointment. He spoke with his secretary for a few minutes, giving me time to settle in a chair and take in the room.

The calm I'd felt only minutes before vanished. Why was I there? I had no idea what I was going to say, or even why I had asked to see Gabri. Was I feeling sorry for myself? Was I looking for relief from the guilt I felt for getting angry with Geoff, then fearing he would die in hospital before I could make it up to him? Was it sheer panic at how swiftly I seemed to be losing Geoff? I knew Gabri only from attending his Mornings with Julian of Norwood study group and working in the homeless program. There was no context for pouring my heart out to him, and I knew that was about to happen. I was mortified and hadn't yet said a word.

Gabri sat down opposite me and said, "Well?"

I said, "My husband . . . "

In that instant I knew why I was there. Losing Geoff was so terrifying it made me shake. I broke into trembling, gulping sobs. Through my tears I saw a Picasso print leaning against the wall and tried to talk about the artwork instead of Geoff. I couldn't handle losing him, couldn't bear to think about it, much less express it. Nor could I own up to the rage I sometimes gave in to, and the dreadful fear that wracked me when I left the house or went into another room where I wasn't near Geoff. Those feelings of anger and fear were too awful to reveal, even to a priest or to Susan, my close friend of nearly fifty years.

Facing what I knew was inevitable and all too immediate was more than I could stomach. I felt ill, only half hearing Gabri tell me all the things I should already know, trying to find comfort, but aching with sorrow for what I knew was ahead. Geoff was pulling away and I was already losing my connection to him.

One afternoon, as the cold, dreary days of February dragged on, the tense tedium of hospice care recorded in detail on charts in a thick binder, it hit me what my life might be like on my own. I'd finished my work for the day. Bills were paid, my desk cleared, with file folders neatly returned to a wire rack next to the telephone. I looked out my office window to see if the mail had been delivered, but the flag was still up on the box. The clouds had cleared, the sun bright. I picked up my mug of tea and took a walk in the garden, then looked back toward the bedroom.

Karen was sitting next to Geoff, both watching a film on television. She would be leaving in less than an hour. As I took in the quiet scene, a burst of sunlight flared against the windowpane, an opaque veil blotting out their images with a suddenness that made me gasp. Gone. Empty. Alone. With a racing heart, I hurried back inside to be with Geoff.

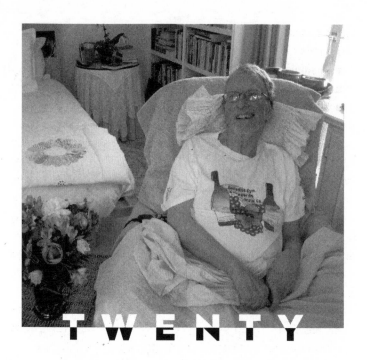

TWENTY

"IN THE STILL OF
THE NIGHT"

February 28, 2011—*I have to go to London, can't put it off
any longer. Paul is very ill, leaving the Cottage unattended. It's
time to give it up once and for all. I'm scheduled to leave in a
matter of days. I've bought food, prepared meals, left written
instructions and still wonder if I'll actually be boarding a flight.
If I am to make a quick trip, now would be the time, but only if*

Geoff's condition remains stable. I try not to think too much about going because I feel guilty about my eagerness and hope it doesn't show. It's a trip I have to make, but also want to make. I need to get away. How odd, when it's inevitable that the time is coming when I won't have these considerations . . . With that thought comes a pang that knocks the breath out of me.

Our friend Paul, who ran a boutique hotel in our London neighborhood and managed the Cottage for us, was in an isolation ward in hospital, his disease terminal. I talked to Ben about the situation, although there was little to discuss. Our beloved cottage had become a liability for us, a circumstance we could no longer ignore. It was time to give it up. I could deal with the pressing matter more readily than Ben, so I made arrangements to return to London.

My brother Orlyn called. "I'm sitting here looking at an itinerary on my computer screen. I could be there Saturday and stay while you're gone."

"No, you don't have to do that, really. It's expensive. You can't take the time from work."

"I was thinking that if you're out of the country you should have a family member on hand with Geoff . . . "

"But I shouldn't even be going. He's really not well . . . "

"I just pushed the button. My flight's booked."

I was relieved Orlyn would stay with Geoff the five days I would be gone. He could arrange for me to Skype daily with Geoff. He could relieve Karen, and if anything went terribly wrong, he would know what to do. He was also a good cook.

March 1—*Hard. The whole day has been hard. The hospital bed was delivered. Everyone said it was time. Geoff would* be more comfortable. I would get more sleep. The health care workers would be happier. He could be turned. He would have support sitting up. There would be railings to protect him from falling out of the bed. Smiles all around—even from Geoff, who had whispered he wanted a hospital bed. But I knew how much I would miss having him next to me. I held him close last night, knowing the bed would be set up today. After his bath, Geoff was eager to be tucked in, grinning at all the tricks his new bed could do. He liked the electric mattress that inflates, deflates to ward off bedsores, and the mechanism that lifts his knees and raises his back. I hate the bed, the green monster that's stolen my husband and makes that terrible wheezing sound as though it's sucking the very life out of him.

Orlyn arrived. I went over instructions with Karen again, then showed my brother where I kept the sealed packet of "emergency" papers, including power of attorney, insurance files and other documents he might need. I spent some private time with Geoff, speaking softly, making sure he understood why I was flying to London. I told him I would be coming back soon, that he would see me on Skype every day.

"Say hi," he murmured, and then I knew he understood where I was going.

"I will. Back soon. I love you." I gave him another kiss.

Orlyn dropped me at the airport and I made my way through security checks in short order. With time on my hands in the departure lounge, I sat in a corner, so torn up I considered canceling my flight. As eager as I'd been to depart, I was suddenly overwhelmed with misgivings. How can I leave? Am I crazy?

Trish picked me up at Heathrow. Beautiful Trish— smiling, confident and welcoming—drove me to their new house in Chiswick, urging me to stay with them rather than go to the London cottage. As soon as I mounted the stairs to their guest room, with its dormer windows and view of chestnut trees, I knew I would be staying in their warm, embracing home for the duration of my trip. Besides, I didn't really want to be by myself in the Cottage, alone with my thoughts and memories.

There was no time for jet lag. The following morning, I shook off grogginess with a cup of strong PG Tips and a brisk walk to the train station. The sky was sullen, threatening a deluge. By the time I reached Sloane Square, the streets were wet and I had to struggle to keep my umbrella from turning inside out in the blustery March wind. I jumped on a 137 bus that careened around Hyde Park toward Marble Arch, my stop.

I marveled again at the changes in my old neighborhood, remembering the sedate bygone days when milk in a bottle was delivered to our front door in the morning along with two newspapers. When I first lived in London, I carried schillings in my pocket and shopped at the neighborhood fishmonger, "Scotch" butcher, greengrocer and bakery. I bought fresh roasted coffee beans and boxes of loose tea from a fragrant shop on the corner, and always stopped in at Dillons bookstore down the street on my way home. My formerly cozy, slightly seedy neighborhood had grown decidedly more upscale over the years, with Madonna living in the next street and former prime minister Tony Blair and his family moving in nearby.

I raced into the new French patisserie for coffee and a croissant to go, checked mail in the entranceway to the Cottage and unlocked the door to the garden. Paul had spruced up the Cottage before becoming ill. A handsome teak table and chairs were set up under the tree in front of the big bay window. The perimeter of the patio was freshly dug for spring planting.

I turned the key in the door and heard the familiar deep-throated sigh as it swung open. As I always did, I paused on the threshold to breathe in the very particular smell of the Cottage, a pleasant herbal, musky fragrance that seemed to meld sage, rosemary and wood fire. It was the smell of the house I'd lived in longest in my life.

The fireplace, which was red brick the last time I saw it, was now painted white. The old Victorian lamps and roll-top desk somehow worked with the new white leather couches and flat screen television. I stood with my coat still buttoned, my umbrella hanging moist and limp in my hand, and had another cry. Geoff was not here with me. This was no longer my home.

I walked around upstairs, poking in empty closets and bureaus, lamenting the missing brass bed that had been replaced with a sleek platform and a mattress smothered in a white duvet. "People like white things," Paul had said. "No brown furniture, no quaint old beds." Gone was the fitted carpet, ripped out to lay down pale new hardwood floors. Recessed lighting, fancy kitchen appliances and a power grid that could handle digital-age electronics had somehow found their way into a cottage built in 1791, despite its Grade II historical listing. Paul had done a good job, but unfortunately he wouldn't be around to fully realize his investment.

I photographed every room in the Cottage, made a

few calls, went through the mail, drank my coffee and left. I realized I hadn't bothered to turn up the heat. I'd never even unbuttoned my coat.

I spent my days taking care of all the business I needed to do regarding the Cottage, and did so at a swift pace. The streets of London, with all its nook-and-cranny twists and turns, are more familiar to me than my hometown in Minnesota. Besides, I could again enjoy walking unencumbered, arms swinging, with no wheelchair to push. I could jump on and off buses, whiz through tube stations, visit friends who lived in places with stairs, and stride across Hyde Park, my face lifted to the chilly mist. I went to the theatre, stayed up late, and every time I realized why I could do so, I'd burst into tears. As I wrote in my journal, inevitably the time was coming when I could do those things whenever I wanted, but I wouldn't have Geoff. The thought was unbearable.

How odd it was to get together with old friends and go places Geoff would have loved. Julian Fellowes, newly minted Lord Fellowes, invited me to lunch at the House of Lords. I arrived early because I didn't want to miss a moment of that amazing experience. After going through a security screening in the reception area, I took my time in the antiquated powder room. I examined everything: the paneled walls, soap dispensers, linens and every ancient fixture. I spent at least a half hour sitting on a leather settee, pretending to read a newspaper while watching the arrivals rush in, shaking out umbrellas, shrugging off the damp cold and greeting each other in bright, modulated tones. Everyone looked important.

I was so engrossed in eavesdropping that I was

startled to hear Emma Kitchener Fellowes' distinctive voice trilling my name. I looked around, once again astonished by her beauty and sheer presence. Towering above me, a glamorous white turban concealing her waist-length chestnut hair, she was full of unnecessary apologies about Julian being delayed on the *Downton Abbey* location shoot, checking the historical accuracy of a tweed jacket. I laughed, because—well, of course that's what Julian would be doing.

She whisked me through corridors of elaborately carved paneling into great halls with decorative ceilings and beautiful floors, my eyes trailing past glorious tapestries and sculptures. Along the way to a cozy bar, Emma pointed out the portrait of her great uncle, Lord Kitchener, and told me she'd "grown up in the Lords," celebrating birthdays and her wedding to Julian. We'd barely ordered drinks before Julian joined us. Off we went to the dining room for typical English fare: roast pork, good claret and glittering conversation.

Squeezed among business meetings, I managed to meet up with other good friends for lunch and tea, including Jo-an and Adrian. I also spent time at the Cottage saying goodbye to it in a loopy, rambling remembrance filled with bouts of tearful laughter. It wasn't the first time that, alone in the Cottage, I'd talked aloud to those thick stone walls! How many times had I used tubs of spackle trying to patch the cracked bedroom wall that had been splintered by a buzz bomb in 1944?

IRA bombs had shaken those same walls in the 1970s, when I'd had to make my way past yellow police tape to the Prince of Wales Theatre near Leicester Square, where I was doing *Harvey* with Jimmy Stewart.

During the infamous coal strikes in the early 1970s, I'd sat in the kitchen reading Agatha Christie by candle-light, drinking cheap port with good cheddar and shivering in layers of sweaters and blankets. The parties, dinners, houseguests and days spent writing on an old Smith Corona at the dining table came flooding back. I recalled the first time Geoff saw the Cottage, his eyes taking in the beamed ceiling, tall bookshelves lining the walls and the cozy wing chairs next to the fireplace. "I feel at home," he'd said.

I also remembered the night we'd danced at the Savoy and then walked home, the night still warm, the streets quiet well after midnight. We'd sat in the garden, light glowing in the cottage windows, sipping Armagnac, talking quietly. We hadn't wanted the evening to end, savoring every moment until Geoff had to leave in the morning.

It was time for me to leave, too. I hugged the walls—and yanked the old chain pull on the World War I vintage toilet before I left. I wouldn't be back in the Cottage again. At the last moment, I'd taken an odd little teapot I knew would fit in my luggage, then looked around one more time. I was ready to say good-bye. I pulled the latch closed and patted the door with a farewell kiss, offering my blessing to the new occu-pants.

Out on the street, I took a lingering look at the bed-and-breakfast next door, once the home of Jennie Churchill. Geoff and I, in preparation for our UCLA Plato course on Winston Churchill, had climbed the circular stairs to photograph his mother's boudoir, still architecturally as it was when she died there in 1921 after slipping on those treacherous stairs in new high-heeled shoes. I was struck by twin thoughts. First: How many hotel guests booked into that room knew it was her boudoir? Second: How could Geoff have climbed those steep, circular stairs only two years earlier?

At the end of each day, I walked from the Chiswick train station back to Trish's house, tired but exhilarated. The first thing I did was boot up Skype to catch Geoff as he finished his breakfast. I was desperately lonesome for him and would call again before going to bed each night, a comfort, but also wrenching because it gave me a true sense of his condition. His face was lean and handsome as ever (*how did he manage it?*), but his hair and beard were bone white. He couldn't speak. His smile was fixed and crooked, but his blue eyes sparkled when he saw my face only inches from his.

Afterward, I'd lie in bed, my chest aching, imagining what he must be suffering emotionally behind those warm, expressive eyes. He never complained, never talked about how he felt even when I gently urged him to open up to me. How could he be so accepting?

I was nowhere near so accepting. I was eager to get home, breaking down because I knew what was ahead. James wrapped his arms around me, comforting me. He and Trish took me to the airport and James walked me to the entrance. I flew Air New Zealand in an airplane only a week old, seated in an economy section, feeling like I was in first class. I had a glass of wine, tried to read, then stared out the window at the sweep of thick clouds much of the way home.

Halfway there, I was seized with terrible anxiety and grew more anxious as the twelve-hour flight dragged on. *What if?* Hadn't I left my mother for a quick trip to

California? Only four days away from her, but it had been four less days with my mother and I'd let her down by leaving. I willed that brand-new airplane to fly at sonic speed, praying, *Get me there before it's too late!*

We touched down and I called Orlyn instantly. All was well. Harry picked me up and I was home within the hour. I raced up the stairs. Geoff was sound asleep. Karen looked exhausted. She said Geoff had become congested, moaned and required turning throughout the night. She and Orlyn had barely slept. After she left and Orlyn turned in, I slipped off my shoes, crawled into the hospital bed and held Geoff close.

The following morning, Harry took my brother to the airport while I stayed with Geoff. Flowers arrived from Carol Dudley, our friend in London. I photographed them on a table next to Geoff. He managed a smile and looked happy, a lovely picture to email back to Carol. I held his hand and told him about my trip, once again describing every amazing moment in the House of Lords. I reminisced about the Cottage and described in detail the changes Paul had made. Geoff looked intently at me, seeming to relish every word, then asked for a malted milk. He got his wish, along with flapjacks for dinner.

That night, I curled next to Geoff in the hospital bed, but awakened, stiff and chilled, in the early light of morning. The mattress inflated, deflated, with a faint rocking sensation, as though the two of us were lying together in a rowboat, a summer breeze skimming across our faces. I shifted in the bed, feeling cool air from the open window on my bare shoulders. The covers had slipped off my back and were bunched up around

Geoff. His eyes were open, radiant blue in the soft light of dawn. His lips moved. I leaned close.

"Malt," he whispered, the word sounding like a quiet yawn.

"Coming up," I whispered.

I released the railing on the hospital bed, slid off the puffy mattress and ran through my checklist. First things first, I adjusted the oxygen tubes and turned on CNBC. Geoff needed to be turned, changed and medicated before I could make him his breakfast, but his own priority was to follow the stock market while sipping a banana-and-blueberry malted milk.

The following week, Dan Levinson arrived from New York to play in a jazz festival. He visited Geoff one afternoon, clarinet case in hand, to give him a private concert. He didn't have to ask Geoff what he wanted to hear. He knew. Dan played "On Green Dolphin Street" and "Invitation," both by Bronislau Kaper, among several other selections.

Geoff's lips moved, mouthing, "Thanks."

"That's okay, I needed to warm up for tonight," Dan said, his voice choked. He took a moment before adding, "How else could I thank you for introducing me to Artie Shaw? I won't ever forget that dinner."

As the following few weeks drew to a close, Geoff grew noticeably weaker and had difficulty breathing. Karen showed me again how to use the nebulizer, a piece of equipment that helped clear his lungs. I filled it with medication, plugged it in and told her I could manage. Before she left for the day, I helped her change Geoff and ease pillows around him. I sat next to his hospital bed, holding his hand, reading aloud a chapter from the Louis Armstrong biography *Pops*. I filled a straw with a bit of water and slid it to the side of his tongue. He choked a bit. I mopped up, comforted him and continued to read.

The nurse made a visit the following afternoon. She told me there were signs indicating Geoff was in an "active phase of dying." I stared at her. He drank a malted milk this morning! He watched the stock market. He smiled when I read him *Pops*.

"Imminent," she said again, "perhaps a matter of days."

She sat at my desk, using my phone to order round-the-clock staff, arranging for a nurse from four in the afternoon until midnight, with another nurse on duty from midnight until eight in the morning. I was complicit in this, even as I felt guilty that I was letting it happen. The rest of the equipment I'd stashed in the guestroom closet was hauled out. The really serious medications I'd hidden in the back of the vegetable crisper were now placed front and center in the refrigerator.

I called my church, reaching Fr. Gabri's assistant to request a pastoral visit. Although Geoff was Catholic, Gabri, an Episcopal priest, had been raised Catholic at Good Shepherd, the same Beverly Hills church Geoff's family had attended. Both he and Gabri had served as altar boys there, decades apart—and both had mothers named Rosemary. That had to count for something.

Even as a full hospice task force was assembling, Tim and David arrived with In-N-Out burgers and chocolate malts. Neither could believe that Geoff and I had never had them before. "If not now, when?" I asked.

The nebulizer did its work. Geoff looked alert, his

eyes lighting up with the smell of burgers wafting into the bedroom. I fed him minute bits of meat and used a straw to drip melted chocolate malt onto his tongue. He smiled, grateful that David and Tim could maneuver him into a chair by the window. While they visited, I poured myself a glass of wine and took a walk in the garden, breathing the sweet smell of night-blooming jasmine. The scare was over. Nothing was "imminent." We'd had our first In-N-Out burger together, and there would be more to come. All was well for the moment and I didn't want to think beyond the present.

After the nurse and I changed Geoff and settled him for the night, I told her she could go home. I also asked her to cancel the night nurse. She hesitated, but obliged after going over the medication schedule with me. I closed the door, feeling at peace alone with Geoff. I held his hand and told him how much he meant to me, that I would love and comfort him as long as he needed me. I read to him until he fell into a deep sleep.

I fell asleep in our bed a few feet away, but awoke to his moans a short time later. His leg was hitched over the railing and he was trying to sit up. "How do I get out of this contraption, damn it?"

"You can't, but I can join you." I gave him medication, removed a thick pillow and crawled into the hospital bed next to him, my arm wrapped protectively across his chest.

In the morning, I tried to feed Geoff soft oatmeal with mashed banana. He closed his lips and turned his head away. Karen arrived and said, "Soon. He's close. Don't try to feed him anymore. It's not good for him now."

The hospice nurse arrived, surprised that I'd discontinued around-the-clock care. Geoff's condition had deteriorated. He had a fever. He was congested and his breathing was labored. She showed me how to give medication slowly, under the tongue. I carefully checked the markings on the plastic syringe, then noticed the label.

"It's morphine."

She saw my alarm. "It'll help his breathing. The Ativan will calm him and help clear the congestion. Don't try to feed him. He's letting you know. He can't swallow and it's painful."

I looked at Geoff, startled to see the deterioration that had taken place in a matter of hours. "You don't have long," the nurse said. "You need more help. He has to be turned more often and he needs breathing treatments to make him comfortable. You can't handle this on your own." She made a call to reinstate twenty-four-hour care.

Fr. Gabri arrived at three o'clock. The medication and breathing treatments had restored Geoff's color. His eyes were clear and he even managed a smile. Gabri told wonderful stories about his mother, Rosemary Clooney, and his childhood growing up on Roxbury Drive. Geoff grew up near Roxbury Park, where he rode his tricycle as a little boy. I reminded Gabri that both had also been altar boys at Good Shepherd Catholic Church, where Geoff served at Elizabeth Taylor's first wedding to Nicky Hilton. I related some of Geoff's stories, but Gabri bested ours by telling about his godparents, Bing Crosby and Billie Holiday. I stood next to Geoff, holding his hand, feeling his response, seeing the laughter in his eyes. Gabri asked Geoff if he wanted last rites. I nodded on his behalf.

Despite having nurses on hand, I still climbed into the hospital bed with Geoff at night, not sleeping but holding him in the dark for a few hours before retreating to the sofa couch in the den. Geoff's stepchildren, Lori and Steve, and various close friends dropped by throughout the week. Several of them, I knew, wanted private time with Geoff. There were thanks to be said, amends to be made. When friends and family members left, I looked at Geoff and wondered how much he'd heard or comprehended. Yet I understood how meaningful those private moments were for those who would go on living after Geoff was gone. I coveted every moment with him myself and knew it wouldn't ever be enough.

Geoff had stopped eating and was unresponsive, but still I wrestled with the terrible thought that I was making a mistake. Who said it's time to let him go? I should feed him. I should give him water. This could be turned around!

The nurses knew what I was thinking. Perhaps I even said it aloud. In any case, each made a point of telling me not to feed him, that his body was not accepting nutrients, that force-feeding would only prolong the inevitable and increase his suffering. He had closed his lips, refusing nourishment. He choked on liquid, even tiny amounts dropped in his mouth through a straw. He had not wanted to be intubated. He'd been adamant about not having a feeding tube. He's choosing his time, I was told.

I stood behind the hospital bed, stroking his face, my own face wet with tears he couldn't see. I spoke softly, my voice low and gentle, masking the pain I felt. In those final weeks, as he pulled away, I reminded myself of what he'd told me when my mother neared her end. "It's her journey. Just be there for her."

I sensed then why I would never have regrets about my trip to London. I felt calm after facing a reckoning I'd dreaded: *How could I ever give up the Cottage, my home most of my adult life?* Yet I had, and I was at peace with the decision. But far more significantly, distance and that brief time away from Geoff had given me perspective. I gained clarity as the last thin veils of hope, fear and denial fell away. I would be able to handle what had seemed beyond imagining.

Holding him close, feeling his warmth, I knew in my bones that my precious time with him would soon be over. Without tears getting in the way, I released myself to the pure sensation of just being with him in his final days.

And, of course, life went on all around us. Email arrived from the London *Sunday Telegraph*, requesting an update on the piece I'd written months earlier. I sat with my laptop in a chair at Geoff's bedside, reading the entire piece aloud to him before emailing it to the *Telegraph*. Finished, I closed the lid on my laptop and looked to Geoff for approval. Even though he couldn't respond, I wanted him to at least hear what I'd written. How I ached to hear his comments!

Saturday, April 16—*I awake before dawn to find the night nurse giving Geoff medication. He looks gaunt, his eyes milky and half-closed. His breathing is quiet and regular. The night nurse tells me that a day nurse is not available. He offers to stay an extra hour and I thank him profusely. I rush to shower, make myself tea and then assist him in changing and cleaning Geoff.*

Suddenly, as Geoff was turned on his side, he

coughed and his eyes flew open, gloriously blue and bright. He seemed surprised to see me.

"Hi," I said, a bit bashfully, as though we were meeting for the first time. Then, feeling the warmth of his gaze, I mouthed, "You are the handsomest man I ever met. I love you."

The nurse, reluctant to leave me on my own, carefully went over the meds to make sure I understood how much I should administer at each interval. By sunup, the nurse had left. I sat next to Geoff, holding his hand. His eyes were closed, his breathing regular. I picked up *Pops* and read the final chapters to him.

Several hours later, the doorbell rang. "Oh, they've sent someone anyway," I said to Geoff, then went downstairs to open the door.

A thickset woman wearing nurse's scrubs stood on the doorstep. Without catching her name, I hurried back up the stairs. She followed me to his bedside, but then did little more than stand and gaze at him. "He doesn't need medication. You can tell by looking."

I asked her to check his temperature, but she didn't have a thermometer. "I leave them everywhere, so I stopped buying more." I asked her to help me shift him in bed and readjust the pillows. "But why disturb him when he's sleeping so nicely?" she said.

She was unnervingly placid. Her voice was listless and there was a vacant look in her eyes that aroused my suspicions. "You're right," I agreed. "We'll let him sleep."

"Do you have any coffee?" She looked at me eagerly. "I could sure go for some."

Seeing this sudden spurt of animation, it dawned on me that she could be an imposter angling to be left alone to scavenge for valuables and drugs while I was out of the room. I wanted her out of my house. "Good idea. Come down with me so we can talk."

"Someone should stay with him."

"He'll be fine. Let's go," My manner was firm, but I'd begun to quake inside. After a moment's hesitancy, she turned toward the stairs. Keeping some distance between us, I followed her down and opened the front door. "Thank you for coming. Goodbye."

Without a word or backward glance, she walked out the door. I watched until she reached the street, then closed the door, my fingers trembling as I turned the lock.

I went back upstairs and stood at Geoff's bedside, still feeling shaky. "Wow, what did you think of that? Do you believe it?" I half expected him to laugh. It was the sort of absurdity he would appreciate. But then, hearing only silence and feeling a bit lightheaded, I looked around for some sign that the stranger had actually been there. Had I imagined it? Or had I just experienced my own Princess Di encounter?

I made coffee, then sat next to Geoff, my cell phone within reach, a pile of scrapbooks at my feet. I placed one of them on the bed and begin paging through it, commenting brightly on long-ago dinner parties and vacation trips. How young we looked, how carefree! "Remember this?" I said over and over as I flipped pages, running my fingers over snapshot memories of our St. Patrick's parties, Christmas gatherings and vacations. Occasionally I got up to change music, selecting his favorite Artie Shaw and Benny Goodman CDs.

I stroked his chest and held his hand, speaking softly. He looked peaceful, his breathing regular, but he seemed warm. I put cold cloths on his forehead and chest, then gave him medication. The moment the syringe touched his lips, his mouth moved hungrily. I slowly squeezed the plunger under his tongue, worried I'd waited too long to give him pain medication.

Minutes later, shortly after five o'clock, the doorbell rang. John, a slim, young hospice nurse I hadn't met before, stood on the doorstep. He was dressed in navy blue scrubs, with a stethoscope slung around his neck and a scarf tied around his forehead. His eyes were warm, intelligent, and he looked as though he'd probably be packing a thermometer. I realized I was glad to see him. I brought him up to date while he checked Geoff's vitals. He winced when I told him I'd delayed giving him medication because he looked too peaceful.

"I think we should make up for it now. His temperature is 103. But first I need to turn him over a bit and I want you to stay with me. Sometimes moving a patient like this can precipitate a rapid change. You should be here."

I understood. Geoff's eyes flew open again as we shifted him. I supported his head, stroking his cheek, as John changed him and gave him medication. When we finished, John suggested I take a walk in the garden.

"Get something to eat. You need a break. Let me look over the papers you have from UCLA, just in case. I'll call you if there's any change."

I went to the kitchen and nibbled a piece of chicken, my first food of the day. Afterward, I walked up to the rose garden and perched on a bench with a view of our bedroom. Through the French doors on the balcony, I saw Geoff lying in the hospital bed, John hovering next to him. A surge of warmth, of well-being and calm, suffused me. Perhaps it was the nourishment and my trust in John—perhaps it was the sensation that Geoff was actually with me in the garden, that the two of us together were observing a scene playing out behind the proscenium of an open window. Minutes passed, shadows lengthened, and an evening chill wrapped around me, but I continued to watch, feeling Geoff at my side.

I was almost unaware that John had stepped onto the balcony. He looked up at me and I knew it was time. While John went into the den, I rebooted the CD player with Artie Shaw and Cole Porter, and then sat next to Geoff. It was six o'clock. I held his hand and lay my head on his chest, my fingertips on his cheek. His breathing changed, becoming more rapid. He was panting for breath. I looked up. His eyes were open, brilliant blue and clear. He looked so young, his skin taut, smooth and very pale. I stroked his cheek, then cradled him in my arms. For more than an hour—a lifetime, really—I held him close, listening to music.

"Do you remember? The orchestra played that piece when we danced at the Savoy?" Looking into his eyes, I hummed a bit of "Night and Day." "We danced to this and fell in love, remember?"

My lips to his ear, I whispered, "No tears. Not now. I'm with you as long as you need me. Then go and find a place for us." Cradling him in my arms, we could've been dancing cheek to cheek at the Savoy. "Thank you, darling. Thank you. Thank you . . . "

I felt him slip away. His breathing stopped. I looked across at John. "I think . . . "

"Yes." He looked at his watch. It was half past seven and night had fallen. "Please take as long as you like with him. I can make the calls."

I kissed Geoff's forehead, smoothed his hair and let him go where I couldn't follow. He grew cold, his face stony, but still playing was Artie Shaw and the music of Cole Porter, and the lingering memory of being wrapped in Geoff's arms dancing at the Savoy on a warm midsummer's evening.

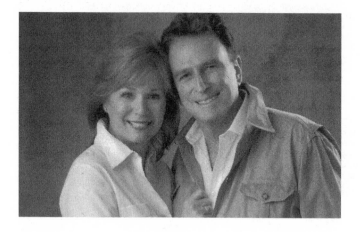

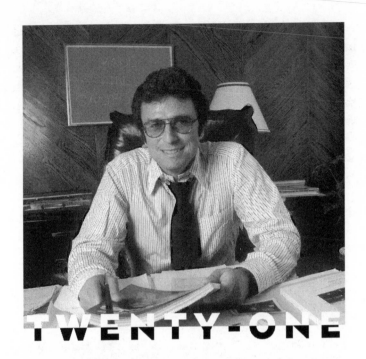

TWENTY-ONE

"EV'RY TIME WE SAY GOODBYE"

The business of death took place in an orderly fashion. After lingering at Geoff's bedside, trying to comprehend the profound chill of his absence, I kissed his cooling cheek and left the room. John, the hospice nurse, took over while I made a few calls, first to Geoff's stepchildren, then UCLA.

"If I'm going to be a guinea pig, let's go all the

way," Geoff had said, agreeing to donate his remains to medical research.

Steve, Geoff's stepson, arrived within minutes. Gil and Miranda, who happened to be driving by our house, stopped in just as Lori, Geoff's stepdaughter, arrived. I took them all in to see Geoff. The bedroom seemed very empty and silent as we approached his bedside. John had purged the side table of registered narcotics and other medications and turned off all the equipment, most noticeably the heaving mattress on which Geoff lay, a still effigy of the man I'd known and loved.

I fielded calls from obituary writers at *The New York Times* and the *Los Angeles Times*, realizing that one of Geoff's close friends I'd called had notified them.

Meanwhile, I also dealt with the missing paperwork confounding UCLA's computer system. "Figure it out or forget it," I told the hapless clerk manning the switchboard, knowing they would have to retrieve his body quickly or not at all. But then I managed to reach Yvette Bordelon at home and she immediately made the necessary arrangements.

Gracious friends offered to spend the night with me. "You shouldn't be alone," I was told, but that's all I wanted. I needed to be alone, to sob and make all the loud, ugly sounds I'd managed to contain.

I awoke in the early morning hearing a faint rustling sound, then opened my eyes to see the hospital bed, its puffy green vinyl cover quivering slightly with a gentle wheezing sound. Had the UCLA transport team accidentally turned the motor back on? I got up and turned it off, then lay on the hideous mattress, screaming, "Come back. Just, damn it, come back!

Susan and Connell took me for Sunday lunch. Afterward, I arrived home to find florist deliveries on my doorstep. I unlocked the front door, looked at the empty lift chair and sat on the stairs, blood pounding in my skull, deafening me in the terrible empty quiet. The house was so frighteningly silent.

I jumped when the doorbell rang. The last thing I wanted was to see anyone, but I opened the door to find Candy standing on the threshold. She'd stopped by after church and was holding another flower arrangement a deliveryman had just brought. I sat back down on the stairs, crying as Candy offered comfort and made tea. Recently widowed herself, she understood my sobbing lament. "Come back, damn it! Just come back!"

On Monday morning, the driver from the hospice facility knocked on my door bright and early. He'd come to haul away all the equipment, most gratefully the hospital bed with the slime green mattress. I worked at my desk as he disassembled the bed, but looked up when I saw him appear in the doorway of the den shaking an electrical plug at me.

"See this? See?" He glowered, his dusky face stern. "He coulda been electrocuted! You didn't see that the electrical cord was caught in the metal lift? With that mechanism going up and down, your husband coulda been crisped, know what I mean? Dead!" He snapped his fingers. "Just like that!"

"He is dead," I said calmly.

"But not like that! It's not the way you want to go."

I agreed it wasn't. Then it occurred to me how frequently Geoff and I had shared that hospital bed. With an inadvertent press on the remote control we could've gone up in smoke together. I began to laugh. "Just wasn't meant to be, I guess."

"You gotta be more careful." He shook his head, wound the electrical cord in his hand and went back to work.

Geoff would've howled with laughter. For my part, I never did trust that bed.

The business of death does take a holiday, in our case Passover and Easter. Burials ceased for the duration. The sanctuaries were booked. Anyone not involved in the religious end of things was on spring break, bound for Hawaii or Florida, and that included any medical personnel in charge of autopsies. Geoff's organs were harvested, as he had willed, and his brain was dispatched to the PSP research center, but what remained of his body would not be dealt with for nearly two weeks.

On a Tuesday morning, Bridget drove me to the mortuary. I'd packed up Geoff's best suit, shoes, Turnbull & Asser shirt, favorite tie I'd given him and a spanking new set of underwear and socks. I might have thought I was prepared to make decisions, but everything the funeral director said to me I heard through a fog. Fortunately I had Bridget with me, who fielded every assault on what she knew I had in mind. One needs an advocate in these situations, and Bridget was mine. Afterward, she took me for breakfast at the Beverly Hills Hotel coffee shop—and, yes, libation with eggs is recommended after a trip to a mortuary.

April 23—*Easter morning, staying the weekend with Susan and Connell in their beautiful beach house. I awaken early, not quite six a.m. It's drizzling outside, the beach and sky a* unified gray. I make coffee. It's silent, except for the cawing of birds and steady wash of ocean on the beach. I discover my piece has been published in the London Sunday Telegraph and read it online. It's beautifully edited, and that brings on a fresh flood of tears. Geoff would have loved reading it.

I walk on the beach, thinking about Geoff, of course. I walk perhaps a mile, not quite realizing that I'm both talking to Geoff and about him. In that time, the remembrance forms in my thoughts. I know what I will say at his memorial. Of course I'll do the eulogy—how else will I make it through the service? As I near the house, my cell phone rings. It's my old friend Rob Wolders, a widower himself. "Sundays are the hardest," he tells me, and we chat. Before driving home, I take Susan and Connell for brunch. I get back to find even more flowers on my doorstep.

April 25—It's Tuesday and I meet with Fr. Gabri to plan the memorial service. He asks me who will do the remembrance and I tell him I will, wondering if he thinks that's odd and if I can handle it. All he's seen me do is cry. We assign the readings and prayers to my brothers, Orlyn and David, my nephew Tom, and Geoff's stepson, Steve. Because of the obits and tributes, we could have a sizable crowd of old friends and colleagues—Geoff would want to be in the thick of it, seeing everyone.

Why do I have so much time on my hands? I go home and walk around the garden. Shouldn't I be busy making calls? Shopping for food? I've had so many offers of help, but if anyone helped me I would have nothing to do! The memorial luncheon will be at my women's club, and my book club friends will provide desserts. David, of course, will organize the catering, and Tim will help. I know I should be doing something, but I can't think what. I've put more effort into planning dinner parties! Why is everything so easy? I move too quickly, everything done too fast. Perhaps everything was more taxing and complicated *because I was taking care of Geoff. I was a caregiver. Now I'm not. I decide to bake oatmeal cookies.*

My family arrived the morning of the funeral, a graveside service held at Holy Cross the day before the memorial at All Saints. Harry did the airport runs, picking up Tom and Barb, who arrived from Rhode Island sometime after midnight. In the morning he picked up David, Kari, Orlyn and Marit, who arrived on a flight from Minneapolis, and took them directly to the cemetery. I stood in my driveway wearing a twelve-year-old black suit Geoff loved and holding an armload of flowers from my garden, waiting for Bridget to pick me up. We were going early so I would have time alone with Geoff before the others arrived.

I approached the casket slowly, shyly. Geoff didn't look at all like himself; shrunken, his face stern. His suit looked as though it belonged to someone else. Did he see my disappointment? I tried not to show it. But then, he'd had a full autopsy, his brain shipped to a lab in Florida. Why would he look like Geoff? I touched his forehead, spoke softly, and the longer I stood at his side the more I saw in him my Geoff, my husband.

Family and close friends arrived, twenty of us in all. I met the good-looking Irish priest, who was included in the mortuary package, and suspected he moonlighted as an actor. He spoke in a thick brogue, his voice folksy and mellifluous, perhaps channeling Bing Crosby, who was buried in a nearby plot. His showy performance was immensely pleasing and Geoff would have loved it.

As everyone visited together at the gravesite, I stepped aside to answer my vibrating cell phone. It was a credit card company telling me they'd been informed

Geoff Miller, the primary name on a joint account, had died and the card was therefore canceled. Charges I'd made for funeral expenses had been denied. Orlyn caught my eye and, seeing the look on my face, asked if anything was wrong. I shook my head. Of all the "wrong" things I was dealing with, this was an issue I could handle—*but damn the timing!*

Without much effort, it seemed I'd prepared quite a good lunch. We sat around the long table in the garden, listening to an Artie Shaw CD and the gentle splash of the fountain on the ivy-covered wall. Candy, who'd attended the funeral with her son, was instructed not to lift a finger. But once friends left, my family members did what Norwegians do for leisure: make themselves useful. Instead of taking naps or lying by the pool and reading, they pulled on jeans and tee shirts to scavenge the house for odd jobs to do.

My brother David, who is blind, stood for some time listening to the splash of the fountain before determining why it leaked. He then set about fixing it, no great feat for a man who does fine carpentry and hand built his own log cabin on a remote island in Lake Superior. Orlyn and Tom completely disassembled the stair chair and railings, encasing the heavy equipment in sheets of plastic and storing it in a space in the garage. My sisters-in-law gave me a hand in the kitchen.

Had my family not all pitched in to clean the basement (yes, really!), we would not have stumbled across boxes of sound recordings that had been stored behind the stairs long before Geoff and I married. I did not know the cartons were there, and I think Geoff had forgotten about them. Among many vintage jazz records, we also discovered a treasure trove of homemade acetate recordings and reel-to-reel tapes, some of it disintegrating with age, dating back to Geoff's childhood.

Through a friend of Dan Levinson's, I found a technician who was able to make CDs so I could hear twelve-year-old Geoff talking to his parents and brother, Ed, on Christmas Eve 1948. His parents had both died years before I met Geoff, and I'd never heard their voices. What a delight to hear his mother, Rosemary, chatting brightly over the clink of cutlery on china at the dinner table, speculating whether it would be "Frank or Bing up in the choir loft singing" at the midnight Christmas service at Good Shepherd. How wonderful to listen to tapes Geoff made of jokey conversations with high school pals and frat house buddies at UCLA. What a shame I hadn't found these boxes earlier so Geoff could have heard these recordings! Hearing his voice again, strong and youthful, was a precious gift I'll always cherish.

Thanks to the family trait known as "paint scraping for fun," there were no loose hinges, squeaky handles or Tupperware drawers that needed sorting by the time the sun was setting. To curtail the mending, fixing and heavy lifting for the day, I called Kay and asked her to please invite my family for cocktails so they'd clean themselves up and relax. Afterward, we returned home to eat the chicken potpie Mari Edelman had dropped off.

I awakened early, but not earlier than my family. A second pot of coffee had been brewed and Tom's wife, Barb, was sitting at her computer conducting a conference call at the breakfast table. We arrived at the church early, too, only to find Fr. Gabri dressed in a work shirt and blue jeans, setting up the altar. In his special way,

Dan Levinson thanked Geoff again by returning with a fellow musician, pianist Peter Yarin, to play at the memorial service. Phil Wright, a jazz pianist and family friend, also played at the reception.

With Dan and Peter at the altar warming up, and my family pitching in to help Gabri, it began to feel like a tech rehearsal in summer stock. I checked sound at the lectern, then ran through the order of the service with Orlyn, David, Steve and Tom. With showtime only minutes away, I looked up to see my high school boyfriend, Rob Larsen, who'd flown in from the East Coast, walking down the aisle to greet me.

"You're here!"

"I told you I'd be."

I gave Rob a hug and invited him to join my family at home for dinner that night. Then I looked around at all the other arrivals and began greeting Geoff's colleagues from the magazine, his pals from grade school, high school and college, and a few old girlfriends, as well—and how he would have loved it all. I looked at Fr. Gabri, who I knew would have my back through it all, and he signaled the start of the memorial service.

I was so proud of my brothers, in particular David, who had memorized his passage and walked to the lectern holding Orlyn's arm. Steve, who'd known Geoff from the time he was six years old, and Tom, who had sailed Geoff around the Statue of Liberty and recovered his beloved cap from the waters of the Hudson River, read scripture. Aside from two Cole Porter pieces, Dan also played Maurice Ravel's "Pavane for a Dead Princess," a piece Geoff had specifically requested for his memorial service and lamented that it had not been played at Princess Di's funeral.

That evening, after the reception at the Beverly Hills Women's Club, a contingent of close friends and family gathered in the upper garden for dinner our chef friend, David, cooked on the grill. We talked late into the night, all of us sharing remembrances of Geoff. As the air grew cooler, I told everyone to go into Geoff's closet and find something warm to put on. "And please take it home with you. I want to see you wearing these things again and again . . . "

Time. Suddenly I had so much of it. I tried to take everything a day at a time, wading through the mountain of onerous "widow work" that arrived in thick bundles with every mail delivery. Would I ever have enough death certificates on hand to satisfy everyone who seemed to require one?

It became obvious to me that I had to learn how to deal with the unstructured time that I suddenly had in abundance, and which felt like both a fearsome burden and a source of guilt. I'd excised so many things from my daily life in order to be on hand for Geoff, yet reinstating some of those activities didn't feel appropriate. I'd never been one to race around being busy for busy's sake, but in caring for Geoff I'd effectively grasped how to just be, to stay present and allow life to unfold. It also occurred to me how focused I'd been during the stolen parcels of time when I could write. Now that I had an excess of time, unlimited and unencumbered, could I find the same value in it? My life had changed. It was not going to be what it was and it was up to me to redefine it.

In the late afternoon, I'd step away from my desk and deal with another onerous task: eating. As much as I enjoy cooking, I just didn't want to make dinner for one and eat it while watching the evening news. No, thank you. I was one step away from eating a quick stir-fry out of a skillet over the sink when I discovered happy hour. It soon became my habit to go for a long walk in the late afternoon and head to one of my favorite restaurants, the ones Geoff and I had once enjoyed going to, for their happy hour menu. Often I'd arrange for various friends to join me, and these get-togethers soon became my social life, a quiet, convivial time when I just stopped and enjoyed companionship the way I had with Geoff. It was possibly the most positive new discovery in my life.

Meanwhile, I could feel Geoff working overtime, pulling strings. How else to explain the rush of activity, with so many things we'd talked about coming to fruition in those first few months following his death? After years of delay, Tim Burton had commenced filming *Dark Shadows* in England, with Johnny Depp playing the role of Barnabas Collins. Four of us from the original series were invited to play cameos. Jonathan Frid (Barnabas), Lara Parker (Angelique), David Selby (Quentin) and I (Josette/Maggie Evans) were flown to London in late June to film at Pinewood Studios.

After a tour of the back lot, where the town of Collinsport had been recreated, with shops lining cobblestone streets and fishing boats bobbing in a harbor, we visited the lavish interior sets of the Collinwood mansion. A magical moment occurred when Jonathan came face-to-face with Johnny Depp, costumed and in character as Barnabas Collins. Jonathan scrutinized his makeup and said, "I see you've done the hair," commenting on the signature spiky locks he'd originated some forty-five years earlier.

"We're doing things a little differently," Johnny said. Then he and Tim Burton, both fans of the original series, said, "But we wouldn't be here without you."

It was a bittersweet journey in every respect. As delighted as the four of us were to be working together again, we were hovering on the fringes of an extravagant production that had nothing to do with us. For our beloved Jonathan, crotchety and forgetful, it would be his last venture in front of a camera. He would pass away before the film's premiere.

For me, it also meant an unexpected quick return to London after saying farewell to the Cottage only months earlier. I did not go back for another visit, although I still had a set of keys in my handbag. It would be empty now, ready for new occupants, and I didn't want to see it. But I walked familiar streets, finding reminders of Geoff everywhere in the places we'd been together—and, of course, in the eyes of good friends.

One evening, I joined a group of old mates for dinner, and as we sat down at the table one of them looked around, genuinely bewildered, and asked, "How come we're only five tonight?"

"Because Geoff couldn't make it," I said. We all laughed, unselfconsciously as close friends can, and someone else said, "Oh, of course. I knew something wasn't right."

I arrived back in Los Angeles in the early afternoon, tired from a long flight, and went straight out to the garden. After heavy rains and warm weather, the hillside was blooming with an abundance of roses, freesia and hydrangea. I cut flowers until my basket was full, then transferred the blooms to a bucket of water to take to the cemetery. On my way out the door, I picked up a small photo album laying on the piano and tucked it into my pocket.

I knew Geoff was not really there, but the cemetery provided a designated meeting place. Walking across the spongy grass, I looked down the slope at the long line of gravestones. They were uniform in size, but like a row of identically built tract houses that eventually take on their own character, each marker had shifted, settled and aged in its own space. Geoff's headstone, too, was settling in, skewing upward on one side, its opposite corner bordered with a tendril of curly leaves.

The sod was smooth over his grave, the earth healing. I kneeled on a straw mat and arranged the flowers, then buried my face in the perfumed mass, feeling so raw and torn I could barely breathe. Why could I only picture Geoff as he was when he lay dying, a time so brief in all our years together? I tried to imagine him sitting on the grass beside me, paging through the album with its snapshots of picnics, hikes, dinners in the garden, travel in faraway places. I wanted to picture Geoff as he was in a snapshot, striding toward me in his blue jeans and safari jacket, youthful and handsome, his hair dark and curly. I picked up another photograph of the two of us at a gala event—how I'd love to walk another red carpet with him, holding hands and enjoying the spectacle swirling around us.

Next to that picture was a close up of Geoff wearing a gray tee shirt, holding a martini, his eyes looking straight into mine, his gaze solemn and intimate. I couldn't remember when that shot was taken, but I knew that look. I held the picture for a long time, absorbing that wave of love captured on film, then felt a chill brush across my shoulder. Night was falling.

"Let's go home," I said. I picked up my straw mat and the empty bucket and headed toward my car. "C'mon, Geoff. It's getting late. Come home with me."

Days later, I cleared out a desk drawer and came across a notebook Geoff kept until two years before he died. I flipped the pages and saw the progression, his bold handwriting deteriorating to a scrawl before it stopped entirely. Was I aware at the time? How long did it take me to realize he couldn't open an envelope or write his name? Was I kind enough? Do I regret my moments of impatience? Of course!

I saw my own humanness reflected in a close friend, whose longtime companion was navigating his first day off crutches after breaking his leg. He moved unsteadily to the dinner table and sat down, then looked up at my friend to ask for some water. She was pouring wine. He asked again and she gave him a sharp look and snapped, "You can see I'm busy."

I winced, thinking of the times I was impatient with Geoff eating too slowly. I would hold the spoon and make a small sigh waiting for him to open his mouth. If only I could take moments like those back.

I wish I had another chance, Geoff. I wish it so much, but I don't. And if I had that chance, I'm not sure that with all my good intentions it wouldn't be exactly as it was. I'm so sorry. Forgive me. I need to know that you do.

That sorry lament was on my lips each time I returned to the cemetery and sat at Geoff's graveside. My grief seemed to be escalating, not subsiding. Too soon! Come back! Waves of despondency knocked the breath out of me. I couldn't shake the gnawing guilt and remorse that reason told me was overblown and unwarranted. Yet I wanted to feel his presence, to have one last chance to connect. In my darkest moments, speaking harshly to tufts of sod and a cold marble headstone, I realized what I wanted to hear was that he loved me to the end, that my slights and failings had been forgiven. What I heard was "malted milk," not the endearments I'd longed for as he pulled away on his final journey. I knew better, but it still cut deeply.

"It's foolish of me, I know," I told the bristly grass covering his grave. "But just give me a moment when I feel we're together again the way we once were."

I got my wish sometime later, quite unexpectedly and in a distant place, when my friend Suzanne joined me on an adventurous trip to China. At the tail end of a three-week tour that began in Beijing and included a cruise on the Yangtze River, we arrived in Shanghai. On our first evening, we set out walking from our hotel to visit the magnificent Fairmont Peace Hotel, a masterpiece of Art Deco design. I could only imagine Geoff's thrill at seeing the incredible lobby and then having a drink while listening to music in the Jazz Bar— certainly an occasion for a martini!

Afterward, Suzanne and I walked along the glittering streets, taking a circuitous route back to our hotel that zigzagged well off the main thoroughfare. We had no idea where we were, but I was irresistibly drawn down a side street, where I spotted a placard advertising happy hour.

"My kind of place," I said with a laugh, then looked up and saw that it was a restaurant and bar called the House of Jazz and Blues. The grand entrance, with its dark varnished wood, was decorated with vintage Jazz Age posters and memorabilia. Beyond the crowded bar was a tightly packed room with stained-glass windows and a band playing Hoagy Carmichael's "Stardust," one of Artie Shaw's memorable numbers. If only Geoff could be there! Then I realized he was.

My eyes traveled the length of the bar, sensing that somewhere in the crowd I'd spot him in his safari jacket and Italian cap, absorbed in the music and drinking a martini. I held my breath, waiting for that moment when he'd turn around and see me, amazed and thrilled that I'd found him. I'd seen that look light up his face before when I'd surprised him at Birdland. He'd move aside to make space for me at the bar, then signal James to pour me a glass of white wine. While listening to the Bird-land band, he'd wrap his arm around my shoulders and nuzzle my neck. I knew that feeling and could feel it again in that Shanghai bar, listening to their swing band. The vibrant music embraced me, bringing a flush to my cheeks. Geoff was with me.

Still, arriving back in New York for Christmas, I was struck at not finding Geoff sitting on the couch waiting for me when I walked into the apartment. *You should be here!* I told the sofa. Yet when I plopped down on the cushion where he always sat, I sensed his presence all around me in the stillness.

It felt odd to be out on the streets of New York not pushing a wheelchair. My eyes sought out curbs a block ahead, automatically looking for the handicap slope that wasn't broken, pitted or pooled in water. On the bus, I leapt up to help a man lock his wheelchair in place. An image of Geoff came to mind, bundled in his coat and cap, looking out the window, with me standing next to him, my hand on his shoulder. Geoff got a kick out of the wheelchair lift. I remembered the time when the bus was so crowded that I sat on his lap and gave him a kiss, making a game of it and bringing a smile to the faces of passengers standing around us.

On New Year's Eve, I dreamed. I hadn't had a dream since before Geoff passed away. I fell asleep well before ten and had the most vivid dream in which I was standing with a pile of luggage in a vast hotel lobby. I looked around for someone to help me, then left my red handbag on top of the luggage and headed for the elevator. I had to get Geoff, but I couldn't manage to assist him and also carry the handbag.

"Don't leave your handbag," I told myself. "Not here. Someone will take it." It was the red handbag I'd bought in Italy, my favorite bag, which was showing some wear because I used it so often. I turned back, telling myself to hang it on my arm—but it was gone! I glanced around the huge lobby, knowing Geoff was waiting for me. I couldn't keep looking for my handbag when Geoff was waiting for me.

Then I awoke to the sound of fireworks. It was midnight. I got up and went to check on my handbag, safe on the chair by the front door. I pulled a coat over my nightie and stepped into boots to walk down to the East River, to the same spot I'd walked a year earlier after putting Geoff to bed. I listened to the drumming sounds of distant fireworks and looked up at the night sky glowing with the waves of bright light splashing behind bridges and tall buildings.

I stood looking out on the river, remembering every minute of our last New Year's Eve: Tim and David, our delicious dinner, watching a DVD of *The King's Speech* and then putting Geoff to bed. I also remembered being overcome with emotion and telling Geoff I was just going out for a breath of air.

I recalled the promises I made to myself that night: *Patience. Kindness ... Treasure the joy of precious moments together.* Somewhere, perhaps from the River House apartments on the corner of my street, I heard the tinkling sounds of a piano playing. I swayed back and forth, quietly humming, imagining leaning into Geoff's shoulder, and recalled the feel of his hands on my arms. It would have to do. It was time to get used to things the way they were, but at least I could picture his warm smile and laughing eyes as he pulled me close.

I miss you. I love you. Take me in your arms and let's dance. One last dance.

RESOURCE GUIDE

When my husband was diagnosed with progressive supranuclear palsy (PSP), a neurological disease for which there is (so far) no cure, I yearned for someone to figuratively take my hand and walk with me through the difficult times I knew were ahead.

Little is known about the cause or treatment of this disease that affects some five to six people per 100,000, a number similar to that of Lou Gehrig's disease (ALS). Only about a third of those afflicted with PSP receive proper diagnosis.

Symptoms begin, on average, past the age of sixty, with slightly more men than women affected. According to the CurePSP Foundation, there is no known geographical, occupational or racial preference. While no one actually dies from PSP, and the progression is considered relatively slow, death from complications of the disorder occurs approximately four to seven years after diagnosis. While Geoff exhibited earlier signs of the disease, our clock officially began ticking in late 2007.

It was immediately apparent to me that my husband would need considerable assistance as the disease progressed, but with so little information available, how could I learn what I needed to know to give him proper care? I wanted to hear truth from someone I could trust, told to me in a way I could understand. I required straight talk from somebody with practical experience, expressed with the warmth of compassion. I needed to face cold, hard facts but also receive encouragement and hope for another day.

I scoured bookstores and the Internet, not only for information on the disease itself, but also for stories from people who had already dealt with the progressive stages of these rare prime-of-life disorders, which include multiple system atrophy (MSA), corticobasal degeneration (CBD) and dementia with Lewy bodies (DLB) (with which actor Robin Williams was posthumously diagnosed). Alzheimer's disease is also often included in discussions of these prime-of-life neurological disorders, which usually involve some degree of dementia.

I wanted to know what to expect and how to deal with the steady decline in motor and cognitive ability from caregivers with fresh experience, who had answers to questions I didn't even yet know to ask. I wish I'd had someone to turn to in those early days before Geoff's official diagnosis, when the first troubling symptoms became apparent. While I had friends, family and faith for comfort, I was on my own when it came to coping with the ever-changing "new normal" in our lives.

Geoff lived almost exactly four years from the time of his official diagnosis, but there were earlier signs of neurological impairment that were bewildering, if not alarming, to us. I shudder now to think of the falls, injuries and emergency room visits that, quite frankly, I looked upon at the time as an annoyance. I'm ashamed to admit how often during long waits for stitches and X-rays I expressed my irritation and impatience.

"You need to pick up your feet, for heaven's sake!"

"Can't you watch where you're going?"

The stumbles and falls that seemed inexplicable at the time were early warning signs of the onslaught of a disease characterized by an inability to focus the eyes. But not knowing that, I chided Geoff for being careless, clumsy or (how I regret this!) "having one too many." One of the most difficult things I had to learn was to hold my tongue in the face of each "new normal." Rather than express my exasperation when he spilled or broke something, I reminded myself that he literally couldn't help that his hands were no longer capable of grasping or letting go.

The day-to-day challenges presented by PSP are daunting. If I learned to be patient and to empathize in the face of my own desperation, I also learned not to hide my emotions behind "busyness." While Geoff required assistance and nursing, and I was the designated caregiver, he also needed the comfort of a loving wife just being there for him. I yearned for the husband who had always taken my arm, reached for my hand and been there for me. It wasn't easy to remain linked to the romance that had drawn us together in the first place. Caregiving is hard in all its many aspects, but ultimately it is the most rewarding gift of a loving relationship.

If I were to distill what I learned about becoming a caregiver, it is to forgive myself for my limitations and be there. A progressive terminal illness is a thing of wild unpredictability. Neither you nor the patient has any idea what the next day will bring, only one of the many things not in your power to predict or control. What you can do is listen, comfort and assist to the best of your abilities. It is what you'll remember and cherish.

Thanks to an early suggestion by one of Geoff's doctors, I kept a journal that provided an almost daily record of PSP's progression, including symptoms, medications and the adjustments we made with each new change. It provided a guide to coping and making the best of things when the worst was yet to be faced, and captured what I learned in the process. I strongly recommend keeping a journal—it was an aid to me at the time and is a source of comfort now.

As you follow your own path with this disease, I hope to offer encouragement along the way and inspire you to make the most of the time you have together with your loved one. I recommend the CurePSP website for a comprehensive guide to resources. The CurePSP website provides facts on specific prime-of-life diseases; current contact information for relevant organizations, research studies and clinical trials; resources for handicap products and equipment; and recommended caregiving publications and family conferences.

CONTACT CUREPSP

curepsp.org

E-mail: info@curepsp.org

30 E. Padonia Road, Suite 201, Timonium, MD 21093

261 Madison Avenue, Ninth Floor, New York, 10016

Phone: (US) 800-457-4777, (Canada) 866-457-4777

ABOUT PROGRESSIVE SUPRANUCLEAR PALSY

curepsp.org

PSP: Some Answers: Answers to frequently asked questions about the disease

A Guide for People Living With PSP, CBD and Other Atypical Parkinsonian Disorders: CurePSP's comprehensive guidebook, containing symptomatic treatment suggestions, situational advice and practical wisdom

PSP: A Primer for the Newly Diagnosed: A fourteen-minute video full of facts from PSP expert neurologist Dr. Larry Golbe, and full of hopeful messages from a person with PSP, his wife, a volunteer and Dr. Golbe.

CLINICAL TRIALS AND RESEARCH STUDIES

It's not easy to remain optimistic after being diagnosed with a disease for which there is no cure, but participating in clinical trials and studies gave Geoff hope and a sense of purpose. By nature, he was not complacent and did not want to give up if there was a chance of finding a treatment that would slow or halt the advance of the disease. With his customary good humor, he told his doctors that he was willing to be a "guinea pig" and signed on for drug trials and research studies conducted at UCLA.

For information about current PSP clinical trials, visit clinicaltrials.gov. ClinicalTrials.gov is a registry and results database of publicly and privately supported clinical studies of human participants conducted around the world.

In addition to participating in clinical trials, Geoff donated his brain for research into finding the earliest clinical markers for the onset of PSP, with the goal of developing treatments to slow or stop the disorder as early as possible. Brain donation is the only way to confirm the diagnosis of a neurological disease, and a prime way to contribute to research into these diseases to find a cure. To arrange brain or whole-body donation, speak to your doctor or get in touch with:

Brain Support Network
brainsupportnetwork.org
E-mail: braindonation@brainsupportnetwork.org
PO Box 7264, Menlo Park, California 94026
Phone: 650-814-0848

SUPPORT GROUPS

Early on, one of Geoff's doctors urged me to attend a support group. I resisted at first, reluctant to have to face what I knew was inevitable down the road. But I soon realized that denial wasn't an option and that it was beneficial to meet other people dealing with the same caregiving issues. Among those participating in the sessions were volunteers who had lost a parent, sibling or spouse to one of these prime-of-life diseases and could offer support, encouragement and knowledge drawn from their own experiences.

CurePSP encourages and organizes activities that foster face-to-face communication, exchange, and interaction of comfort and mutual benefit to group members who are caregivers, family members, friends and persons with PSP, CBD, MSA and related diseases. If you are interested in joining a support group, please send an email to info@curepsp.org.

HOME EVALUATIONS AND THERAPISTS

Progressive supranuclear palsy is characterized by a loss of balance, frequent falls, slurred speech, limited eye movement and difficulty swallowing, all of which present risks and injury. Maintaining safety, comfort and enjoyment of daily life become top priorities for anyone living with a progressive neurological disorder. As a caregiver, I learned that as my husband's mobility declined, we had to modify and equip our home to accommodate each new physical challenge. I also learned that, while my husband often required assistance, it was important for him to maintain his sense of dignity and self-reliance as much as possible, for as long as possible. During the course of his illness, we sought professional assistance in physical, occupational and speech therapy.

American Occupational Therapy Association: aota.org; 301-652-2682. Occupational therapists help improve an individual's ability to perform daily activities and regain skills.

American Physical Therapy Association: apta.org; 800-999-2782. Physical therapists are highly trained, licensed health care professionals who can help patients improve or restore mobility and reduce pain and discomfort.

American Speech-Language Hearing Association: asha.org; 800-638-8255

HANDICAP EQUIPMENT AND AIDS

Handicap equipment aided Geoff's independence and helped him feel safe and in control. I strongly recommend having a professional home evaluation visit to assess your particular handicap needs. We arranged a home evaluation with an expert we met at a support group meeting, who pointed out hazards I was not aware of and suggested devices and products that made caregiving much safer and easier. Following are just a few areas in which we made practical adjustments for my husband's safety and well-being, as well as mine as a caregiver.

Among the first pieces of equipment we installed were grab rails and bars in the shower and bathroom, and a riser for the toilet. The representative also advised us to remove throw rugs and other obstacles that could cause my husband to stumble or trip.

Geoff loved to eat, but as he lost dexterity and had difficulty grasping and releasing his grip, I experimented with various eating utensils. I replaced stemware and cups that had handles with plastic tumblers and used a plate with a deep rim. It also helped to put a plastic box under the plate to raise the plate chest-high, making it easier for him to feed himself. Because Geoff was unable to coordinate using a fork and knife, I served food in bite-size pieces. I avoided soup, salad and kernelled corn and peas that were difficult to eat, and popcorn and fruit with seeds that could cause choking. Among his favorite foods were ice cream, yogurt, pasta, pancakes, enchiladas and any number of other flavorful treats that were easy to eat and swallow. Eventually it was necessary to add a thickening product (such as Thick-It) to liquids to make it easier to swallow and prevent choking.

Mobility was a major issue to contend with because of falls and balance problems. Initially, I supported Geoff by grasping his arm and wrapping my other arm around his waist. As Geoff became less steady, his walking more erratic, I felt less capable of assisting him, particularly with the considerable difference in our height and weight. At one of the support group meetings, I learned how to use a gait belt, a thick strap that buckled around his waist and gave me a secure grip. When he lurched too fast or froze in place, we discovered that singing together released him to move at a steadier pace.

Geoff was able to use a rolling walker until he became too unsteady and began to wobble when he walked. The U-Step Walker is considered the gold standard for PSP patients: ustep.com.

Eventually, we invested in a lightweight transport chair that folded easily for use in the house and when we traveled. For city streets and long walks, we had to use a wheelchair. We also had a chair lift installed when it was no longer safe for Geoff to climb the stairs.

One of the early signs of Geoff's disease was slurred speech. Over time, his voice grew faint and he claimed it hurt to speak. Yet he was outgoing and loved conversing with visitors. At Dr. Bordelon's suggestion, I gave Geoff a ChatterVox voice amplifier that came with a headband and a sponge-covered mic that he nicknamed "the Madonna."

To learn more about handicap equipment and products, visit curepsp.org.

CAREGIVING ORGANIZATIONS

National Alliance for Caregivers: caregiving.org; 800-445-8106

Caregiver Action Network: caregiveraction.org; 800-896-3650

Family Caregiver Alliance: caregiver.org; 800-445-8106

Medicare: medicare.gov

Social Security: ssa.gov/compassionateallowances. Assistance in obtaining disability benefits more quickly

National Organization for Rare Diseases: rarediseases.org

National Institute of Neurological Disorders and Stroke: ninds.nih.gov

National Hospice and Palliative Care Organization: nhpco.org

Home Care Association of America: hcaoa.org

National Association for Home Care & Hospice: nahc.org

International Parkinson and Movement Disorder Society: movementdisorders.org

Progressive Supranuclear Palsy Association UK: pspassociation.org.uk

ACKNOWLEDGMENTS

I must begin by thanking my husband, Geoff Miller. This is his story, after all, and he gave me such tremendous inspiration and encouragement as a writer. I trust he is pleased with what I've written about our journey together.

My deepest appreciation to Dr. Yvette Bordelon for writing a beautiful foreword and for reading my manuscript early on, offering her advice and encouragement. I am so grateful to Yvette and her husband, Dr. Carlos Portera-Cailliau, in the Department of Neurology at UCLA Medical Center, for giving Geoff hope and great personal care during his illness.

Cynthia Manson, my literary agent, and Caitlin Alexander, my editor, have both seen me through *Last Dance at the Savoy* from the beginning. Without their encouragement, support and guidance, I'm not sure I would ever have turned my notes and journal into a book. Nicholas Evans, thank you again for another wonderful cover design. Geoff thought the world of you.

My sincere gratitude to David Kemp, Trisha Caruana and Jaclyn Zendrian of CurePSP for their very valuable assistance to me and for the great work they do on behalf of those afflicted with prime-of-life diseases. I must also thank Robert Baensch for his publishing advice and inside knowledge of caring for someone with PSP.

I'm indebted to my family, the Kringstads, in particular my brothers and their wives, David, Kari, Orlyn and Marit, and my nephew Tom and his wife, Barbara, for their love, devotion and unflagging support. My thanks also to Geoff's stepchildren, Lori Selcer and Steve Selcer.

My heartfelt thanks to my extended family, those friends close to us on a daily basis, who gave me so much support and assistance. Candelaria Aquino, Harry Hennig, Tim Anderson and David Chaparro top the list of those who made our lives possible during Geoff's illness. Ben Martin, how very kind you are! Dan Levinson, thank you for all your help with the book and for being such a great friend to Geoff.

My thanks to Mari Edelman, who knows firsthand what it is to be a caregiver and was always there for me. I could also count on my dear friends Hannah Baldwin, Kimberley Cameron, Suzanne Childs, Sunnie Choi, Joan Evans, Bridget Hedison, Miranda Lipton, Pamela Osowski, Susan Sullivan and Heide Wickes for love and support. Kathy Bennett, you are a terrific critique partner and wonderful friend.

My book club friends, Diana Doyle, Angela Movasagghi, Marian Powers and Raleigh Robinson, and my many friends at the Beverly Hills Women's Club were all a great source of comfort and encouragement.

For their support and many kindnesses, I thank Ann and John Allen, Sir Thomas and Jeannie Allen, Mike Anderson, Joel Baldwin, David Brody, Connell Cowan, John Doumanian, Carol Dudley, Adrian Evans, Lord and Lady Fellowes, Fr. Gabriel Ferrer, James, Trish and Max Golfar, Stuart Goodman, Lew Harris, David Hedison, Jackie Hui, Brian Kellow,

Francoise and Douglas Kirkland, Molly Levinson, Gil Lipton, Marilyn and Victor Lownes, Robert Masello, Leesa Mayer, Tia Mazza, Harry McCormick, Patrick McCray, Stuart and Rebecca Pettican, Kay Pick, Anne Pick and Bill Spahic, Dr. Christine Pickard, Stephen Randall, Marcia Roma, Lisa Seidman, Karen Smith, Gordon Trewinnard, Julian Wasser and Rob Wolders.

ABOUT THE AUTHOR

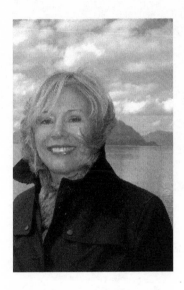

Kathryn Leigh Scott is an author, actress and volunteer spokesperson for the national CurePSP Foundation. She has written several nonfiction books (among them, *The Bunny Years, Dark Shadows: Return to Collinwood, Lobby Cards: The Classic Films* and *Lobby Cards: The Classic Comedies*) and four novels (*Dark Passages, Down and Out in Beverly Heels, Jinxed* and the forthcoming *September Girl*). She grew up on a farm in Robbinsdale, Minnesota, and currently resides in New York City and Los Angeles, where she continues to work as an actress.

Please visit her website at www.kathrynleighscott.com.

Made in the USA
San Bernardino, CA
02 November 2016